$4.80

Physiology

PreTest®
Self-Assessment
and Review

Physiology

PreTest®
Self-Assessment
and Review

Seventh Edition

Edited by

Eileen M. Mulligan, Ph.D.
Assistant Professor
Department of Physiology
Temple University School of Medicine
Philadelphia, Pennsylvania

McGraw-Hill, Inc.
Health Professions Division/PreTest Series

New York   St. Louis   San Francisco   Auckland
Bogotá   Caracas   Lisbon   London   Madrid
Mexico   Milan   Montreal   New Delhi   Paris
San Juan   Singapore   Sydney   Tokyo   Toronto

Physiology: PreTest® Self-Assessment and Review, Seventh Edition
International Editions 1993

Exclusive rights by McGraw-Hill Book Co. - Singapore for manufacture and export. This book cannot be re-exported from the country to which it is consigned by McGraw-Hill.

2 3 4 5 6 7 8 9 0 SEP 9 8 7 6 5 4 3

The editors were Gail Gavert and Bruce MacGregor.
The production supervisor was Gyl A. Favours.
This book was set in Times Roman by Compset, Inc.

Library of Congress Cataloging-in-Publication Data

Physiology : PreTest self-assessment and review, 7th ed. / edited by
    Eileen M. Mulligan.
       p.   cm. - (Basic sciences series)
    Includes bibliographical references.
    ISBN 0-07-051997-8
    1. Human physiology - Examinations, questions, etc.
  I. Mulligan, Eileen M.   II. Series.
    [DNLM : 1. Physiology - examination questions.
    QT 18 P579]
  QP40.P47   1993
  612'.0076 - dc20
  DNLM/DLC
  for Library of Congress   91-38960
                        CIP

When ordering this title, use ISBN 0-07-112983-9

Printed in Singapore

Contents

Introduction

Physiology: PreTest® Self-Assessment and Review provides medical students, as well as physicians, with a comprehensive and convenient instrument for self-assessment and review within the field of physiology. The 500 questions parallel the format and degree of difficulty of the questions contained in Step 1 of the United States Medical Licensing Examination (USMLE) and should be useful for the Foreign Medical Graduate Examination in the Medical Sciences (FMGEMS).

To conform with current USMLE guidelines, all K-type (multiple true-false) questions have been eliminated.

Each question in the book is accompanied by an answer, a paragraph explanation, and a specific page reference to a textbook. A bibliography listing the sources used in the book follows the last chapter.

Perhaps the most effective way to use this book is to allow yourself one minute to answer each question in a given chapter; as you proceed, indicate your answer beside each question. By following this suggestion, you will be approximating the time limits imposed by the board examinations previously mentioned.

When you finish answering the questions in a chapter, you should then spend as much time as you need verifying your answers and carefully reading the explanations. Although you should pay special attention to the explanations for the questions you answered incorrectly, you should read *every* explanation. The author of this book has designed the explanations to reinforce and supplement the information tested by the questions. If, after reading the explanations for a given chapter, you feel you need still more information about the material covered, you should consult and study the references indicated.

Physiology

PreTest®
Self-Assessment
and Review

Metabolism and Endocrinology

DIRECTIONS: Each question below contains five suggested responses. Select the **one best** response to each question.

1. *Paracrine communication* refers to interactions between cells resulting from

(A) direct contact of cells at tight junctions
(B) transmission of mechanical forces via extracellular filaments
(C) release of chemical mediators in localized synaptic junctions
(D) release and diffusion of chemical mediators through extracellular fluid to target cells
(E) release of chemical mediators into blood to act upon specific receptors in distant target tissues

2. Binding of a peptide hormone to its receptor may involve all the following EXCEPT

(A) reversible hydrophobic interactions
(B) allosteric regulation
(C) hydrogen bonding
(D) formation of covalent linkages
(E) coupling with an activity site

3. The supraoptic nucleus of the hypothalamus is believed to control secretion of which of the following hormones?

(A) Antidiuretic hormone (arginine vasopressin)
(B) Oxytocin
(C) Growth hormone
(D) Adrenocorticotropic hormone
(E) Follicle-stimulating hormone

4. Secretion of pancreatic polypeptide is

(A) subsequent to its cleavage from proinsulin in the α cell
(B) a response to both vagal and beta-adrenergic stimulation
(C) the stimulator of release of pancreatic enzymes in response to glucose
(D) inhibited by exercise
(E) none of the above

5. The principal steroid secreted by the fetal adrenal cortex is

(A) cortisol
(B) corticosterone
(C) dehydroepiandrosterone
(D) progesterone
(E) pregnenolone

6. Injection of thyroid hormone into a normal laboratory animal will produce all the following effects EXCEPT

(A) an increase in the rate of oxygen consumption
(B) an increase in the rate of muscle protein synthesis
(C) an increase in the need for vitamins
(D) a decrease in the plasma concentration of cholesterol
(E) a decrease in the rate of lipolysis

7. The effect of insulin on glucose transport is to

(A) permit transport against a concentration gradient
(B) enhance transport across the cell membrane
(C) enhance transport across the tubular epithelium of the kidney
(D) enhance transport into the brain
(E) enhance transport through the intestinal mucosa

8. Compared with the resting state, during prolonged exercise the caloric needs of skeletal muscle are met by

(A) release of free fatty acids from adipose tissue
(B) an increase in hepatic glycogenolysis
(C) an increase in gluconeogenesis in muscle
(D) increased intestinal uptake of glucose and amino acids
(E) none of the above

9. Which of the following statements regarding capacitation of spermatozoa is true?

(A) It occurs in the epididymis
(B) It involves synthesis of androgen-binding protein
(C) It is stimulated by testosterone
(D) It is accompanied by release of acrosomal enzymes
(E) None of the above

10. Removal of the adrenal glands generally has all the following consequences EXCEPT

(A) a tendency to hyperglycemia with decreased insulin sensitivity
(B) poor mobilization and utilization of fatty tissues
(C) poor water excretion by the kidneys and sodium loss in the urine
(D) poor resistance to infection or shock
(E) psychic changes such as depression or decreased alertness

11. Administration of pharmacologic doses of aldosterone to a dog will have which of the following effects upon blood pressure (BP), body weight (BW), and plasma potassium (PP) levels?

	BP	BW	PP
(A)	Increased	Decreased	Increased
(B)	Increased	Increased	Decreased
(C)	Increased	Decreased	Decreased
(D)	Decreased	Increased	Decreased
(E)	Decreased	Decreased	Increased

12. The graph below demonstrates diurnal variation in the plasma level of

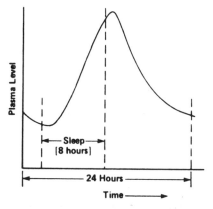

(A) thyroxine
(B) insulin
(C) parathyroid hormone
(D) cortisol
(E) estrogen

13. In the graph below, which shows plasma hormone levels as a function of time, ovulation takes place at which of the lettered points on the time axis?

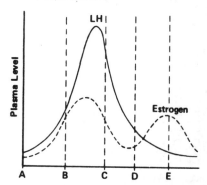

(A) A
(B) B
(C) C
(D) D
(E) E

14. Iodides are stored in the thyroid follicles mainly in the form of

(A) thyroxine
(B) thyroglobulin
(C) monoiodotyrosine
(D) diiodotyrosine
(E) 3,5,3'-triiodothyronine

15. The normal pattern of progesterone secretion during the menstrual cycle is exhibited by which of the curves shown below?

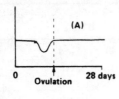

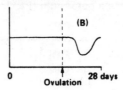

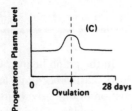

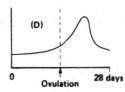

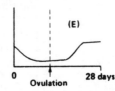

(A) A
(B) B
(C) C
(D) D
(E) E

16. Almost all the active thyroid hormone entering the circulation is in the form of

(A) triiodothyronine
(B) thyroxine
(C) thyroglobulin
(D) thyrotropin
(E) long-acting thyroid stimulator (LATS)

17. Physiologically active thyroxine exists in which of the following forms?

(A) Bound to albumin
(B) Bound to prealbumin
(C) Bound to globulin
(D) As a glucuronide
(E) Unbound

18. All the following are characteristic of hyperparathyroidism EXCEPT

(A) demineralization of bone
(B) formation of kidney stones
(C) hypercalcemia
(D) hypercalciuria
(E) hyperphosphatemia

19. Insulin increases glucose uptake in all the following structures EXCEPT

(A) adipose tissue
(B) cardiac muscle
(C) skeletal muscle
(D) intestinal mucosa
(E) the uterus

20. Hyperglycemia is induced by all the following hormones EXCEPT

(A) epinephrine
(B) thyroxine
(C) ACTH
(D) glucagon
(E) aldosterone

21. Which one of the following hormones is primarily responsible for the development of ovarian follicles prior to ovulation?

(A) Chorionic gonadotropin (hCG)
(B) Estradiol
(C) Follicle-stimulating hormone (FSH)
(D) Luteinizing hormone (LH)
(E) Progesterone

22. The actions of angiotensin II include all the following EXCEPT

(A) direct constriction of peripheral arterioles
(B) promotion of salt excretion by renal tubules
(C) stimulation of aldosterone secretion
(D) inhibition of renin secretion
(E) stimulation of the subfornical organ of the diencephalon

23. All the following statements about somatostatin are true EXCEPT

(A) it inhibits gastrin secretion
(B) it is secreted by the hypothalamus
(C) it is secreted by pancreatic islet cells
(D) it is released following vagal blockade
(E) its effects are prolonged

24. All the following are characteristic of hypothyroidism EXCEPT

(A) bradycardia
(B) decreased metabolic rate
(C) heat intolerance
(D) sleepiness
(E) weight gain

25. In the graph below of changes in endometrial thickness during a normal 28-day menstrual cycle, the event designated "A" corresponds most closely to

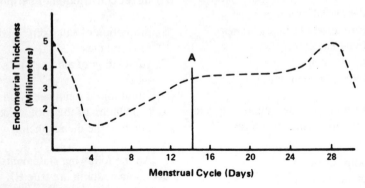

(A) the menstrual phase
(B) the maturation of the corpus luteum
(C) the early proliferative phase
(D) the secretory phase
(E) ovulation

---

26. Goiter (enlargement of the thyroid) can occur as a consequence of all the following EXCEPT

(A) iodine deficiency
(B) pituitary adenoma
(C) Graves' disease
(D) excessive intake of exogenous thyroxine
(E) excessive intake of cabbage and turnips

27. All the following statements about testosterone are true EXCEPT that it

(A) is synthesized in Leydig cells from cholesterol
(B) becomes less active following reduction to dihydrotestosterone
(C) circulates bound to a beta globulin
(D) inhibits luteinizing hormone release at the level of the hypothalamus
(E) is an intermediate in estrogen synthesis

28. In a normal pregnancy, human chorionic gonadotropin (hCG) prevents the involution of the corpus luteum that normally occurs at the end of the menstrual cycle. Which of the curves shown below approximates the level of this hormone during pregnancy?

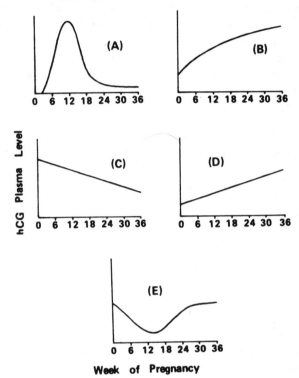

(A) A
(B) B
(C) C
(D) D
(E) E

29. All the following statements about endorphins are true EXCEPT that they

(A) are synthesized as part of a larger molecule that includes the sequence for ACTH
(B) lower the threshold for pain
(C) function as peptidergic neuro-transmitters at many loci within the brain
(D) influence gastrointestinal function
(E) are released from the pituitary during periods of stress

30. Secretion of growth hormone is stimulated by all the following EXCEPT

(A) L-arginine
(B) deep sleep
(C) free fatty acids
(D) growth hormone–releasing hormone (GRH)
(E) hypoglycemia

31. Interaction of insulin with its membrane receptor

(A) affects transmembrane ion transport
(B) inhibits tyrosine phosphorylation in the receptor molecule
(C) reduces cellular glucose uptake
(D) results in enhanced binding of additional insulin molecules
(E) stimulates the synthesis of additional receptor molecules

32. Activation of hormone-sensitive lipase in adipocytes

(A) causes increased hydrolysis of cholesterol esters
(B) is mediated by a cyclic AMP–dependent protein kinase
(C) is prevented by cortisol
(D) is stimulated by insulin
(E) results in accumulation of monoglycerides and diglycerides in adipocytes

33. The basal metabolic rate (BMR) increases with all the following EXCEPT

(A) advancing age
(B) anxiety
(C) body surface area
(D) increased environmental temperature
(E) reduced environmental temperature

34. All the following statements about the uptake of triglycerides into adipose tissue from plasma lipoproteins are true EXCEPT

(A) it is regulated by the activity of lipoprotein lipase
(B) it is decreased by catecholamines
(C) it is increased by glucose
(D) it is increased by insulin
(E) it requires receptor-mediated endocytosis

35. Which of the following is a correct statement about the production of human sperm?

(A) Spermatogonia undergo meiosis
(B) Spermatogenesis occurs in the epididymus
(C) Normally, 10 to 20 million sperm are produced daily
(D) FSH is required
(E) Complete maturation of spermatozoa occurs in 28 to 30 days

36. Functions of the Sertoli cells in the seminiferous tubules include

(A) secretion of FSH into the tubular lumen
(B) secretion of testosterone into the tubular lumen
(C) maintenance of the blood-testis barrier
(D) synthesis of estrogen after puberty
(E) none of the above

37. True statements about implantation of the zygote in the uterus include all the following EXCEPT

(A) it follows dissolution of the zona pellucida
(B) it involves infiltration of the endometrium by the syncytiotrophoblast
(C) it occurs 6 to 7 days after fertilization
(D) it occurs when the embryo consists of approximately 32 cells
(E) it requires secretion of progesterone by the corpus luteum

38. True statements about the development of the wolffian duct system include which of the following?

(A) It is completed during the fifth month of fetal life
(B) It is accompanied by regression of the müllerian duct system
(C) It occurs normally in patients with testicular feminization
(D) It requires the presence of estrogen
(E) None of the above

39. An exceptionally muscular female athlete at an international athletic competition is noted to have increased facial hair and frontal balding. She should be evaluated for all the following EXCEPT

(A) an adrenal tumor
(B) an ovarian tumor
(C) deficiency of 11β-hydroxylase
(D) familial hyperlipoproteinemia
(E) use of synthetic androgens

40. Thyroxine and triiodothyronine are transported in plasma in all the following forms EXCEPT

(A) bound to thyroxine-binding globulin (TBG)
(B) bound to albumin
(C) bound to thyroxine-binding prealbumin (TBPA)
(D) bound to thyroglobulin
(E) as free hormones

41. Thyroid hormones exhibit all the following characteristics EXCEPT

(A) they display a long duration of activity
(B) injected thyroxine raises the metabolic rate within 24 h
(C) they are stored in extracellular sites
(D) they are transported by carrier proteins
(E) they affect the metabolism of most tissues of the body

42. Which of the following statements about iron absorption and metabolism is correct?

(A) About 100 mg of iron is absorbed per day
(B) Iron is absorbed at a rapid rate from the intestine
(C) Iron in the blood is bound to transferrin
(D) Iron ingested in the ferrous state must, in general, be oxidized to the ferric state for absorption
(E) Iron absorption is a passive process regulated by circulating plasma iron levels

43. Melatonin is correctly described by all the following statements EXCEPT

(A) it is synthesized from tryptophan
(B) it regulates skin pigmentation in humans
(C) its secretion is increased by darkness
(D) its secretion is stimulated by norepinephrine from the sympathetic nervous system
(E) reduction of its normal secretion by pineal tumors may cause premature puberty

44. The islets of Langerhans are characterized by

(A) being more plentiful in the head of the pancreas than in the tail
(B) constituting 20 to 30 percent of the weight of the pancreas
(C) containing at least six distinct cell types
(D) having a meager blood supply
(E) producing glucagon and insulin

45. Insulin deficiency leads to increased use of fat as a result of all the following EXCEPT

(A) decreased cellular uptake of glucose
(B) decreased intracellular α-glycerophosphate in liver and fat cells
(C) exclusion of use of glucose except by brain tissue
(D) increased fatty acid release from adipose tissue
(E) indirect depression of use of glucose by excess fatty acids in the blood

46. Secretion of insulin is affected by all the following EXCEPT

(A) blood glucose
(B) Ca^{2+} and K^+ concentrations
(C) 2-deoxyglucose
(D) mannitol
(E) somatostatin

47. Plasma levels of calcium can be increased most rapidly by the direct action of parathyroid hormone on the

(A) kidney
(B) intestine
(C) thyroid gland
(D) bones
(E) skeletal musculature

48. Hyperparathyroidism is reflected in decreased plasma levels of

(A) phosphate
(B) sodium
(C) calcium
(D) potassium
(E) calcitonin

49. Correct statements about human growth hormone include which of the following?

(A) It is synthesized in the hypothalamus
(B) It stimulates production of somatomedins by the liver
(C) Its release is stimulated by somatostatin
(D) It causes a decrease in lipolysis
(E) None of the above

50. Correct statements about progesterone include all the following EXCEPT

(A) it is secreted by the corpus luteum
(B) it is secreted by the placenta
(C) its plasma level is low during the menses
(D) its plasma level remains constant after implantation
(E) its plasma level rises subsequent to ovulation

51. The anti-inflammatory effect of cortisol treatment is thought to be due to all the following mechanisms EXCEPT

(A) decreased capillary membrane permeability
(B) decreased formation of leukotrienes
(C) increased release of pyrogen from granulocytes
(D) inhibition of phospholipase A_2
(E) stabilization of cellular lysosomal membranes

52. In women, estrogens have all the following effects EXCEPT

(A) they facilitate the growth of ovarian follicles
(B) they cause cyclic changes in the vagina and endometrium
(C) they cause cervical mucus to become thinner and more alkaline
(D) they produce ductal proliferation in the breast
(E) they produce glandular proliferation in the breast

53. The basic effects of growth hormone on body metabolism include

(A) decreasing the rate of protein synthesis
(B) increasing the rate of use of carbohydrate
(C) decreasing the mobilization of fats
(D) increasing the use of fats for energy
(E) none of the above

54. Which of the following is true about the actions of glucagon?

(A) It stimulates glycogenolysis in muscle
(B) It inhibits insulin secretion
(C) It stimulates gluconeogenesis in the liver
(D) It inhibits adenyl cyclase
(E) It inhibits phospholipase C

55. One of the most common signs of hypoparathyroidism is

(A) phosphaturia
(B) hypercalcemia
(C) demineralization of bones
(D) hyperexcitability of muscles
(E) formation of kidney stones

56. Cholesterol is the precursor in the adrenal biosynthesis of all the following compounds EXCEPT

(A) aldosterone
(B) cortisol
(C) dexamethasone
(D) testosterone
(E) estradiol

57. Thyroid-stimulating hormone (TSH) increases circulating thyroid hormone levels by increasing all the following EXCEPT

(A) thyroid-binding protein concentrations
(B) proteolysis of thyroglobulin in the follicles
(C) activity of the iodide pump
(D) size of thyroid cells
(E) number of thyroid cells

58. Hormonal changes during normal pregnancy are correctly described by which one of the following statements?

(A) Estriol excretion is greatest just before parturition
(B) Human chorionic gonadotropin secretion is greatest in the third trimester
(C) Human chorionic somatomammotropin secretion is greatest in the first trimester
(D) Oxytocin secretion is greatest in the second trimester
(E) Pregnanediol excretion is greatest in the first trimester

59. Testosterone is synthesized from all the following substances EXCEPT

(A) androstenedione
(B) cholesterol
(C) dehydroepiandrosterone
(D) estrogen
(E) pregnenolone

60. Glucagon characteristically increases all the following EXCEPT

(A) gluconeogenesis in the liver
(B) glycogenolysis in the liver
(C) glycogenolysis in muscle
(D) ketogenesis in the liver
(E) lipolysis in adipose tissue

61. Proinsulin is correctly described in which one of the following statements?

(A) It is a biosynthetic precursor of insulin
(B) It is cleaved by an enzyme on the cell surface
(C) It is a double-chain polypeptide
(D) It is the major form of insulin secreted by the pancreatic β cells
(E) It is more active than insulin on its target tissues

62. The actions of insulin include

(A) converting glycogen to glucose
(B) stimulating gluconeogenesis
(C) increasing plasma amino acid concentration
(D) enhancing potassium entry into cells
(E) reducing urine formation

63. The secretion of ACTH is correctly described in which of the following statements?

(A) It shows circadian rhythm in humans
(B) It is decreased during periods of stress
(C) It is inhibited by aldosterone
(D) It is stimulated by glucocorticoids
(E) It is stimulated by epinephrine

64. Which one of the following statements concerning the conversion of thyroxine (T_4) to triiodothyronine (T_3) is correct?

(A) It occurs primarily in the thyroid gland
(B) It is the primary pathway for inactivation of T_4
(C) It is increased during starvation
(D) It precedes many of the physiologic effects of thyroid hormone
(E) None of the above

65. Male hypogonadism could be produced by a lesion in all the following sites EXCEPT the

(A) testes
(B) pituitary gland
(C) pineal gland
(D) hypothalamus
(E) globus pallidus

DIRECTIONS: Each group of questions below consists of lettered headings followed by a set of numbered items. For each numbered item select the **one** lettered heading with which it is **most** closely associated. Each lettered heading may be used **once, more than once, or not at all.**

Questions 66–72

For each hormone listed below, select the statement that best describes its mechanism of action.

(A) Binds to cell surface receptors and stimulates production of cyclic nucleotides in the cytoplasm

(B) Interacts with a cytoplasmic receptor, then localizes in the nucleus and directs protein and nucleotide synthesis

(C) Binds to cell surface receptors and then activates intracellular processes by a mediator other than cyclic nucleotides

(D) Interacts with a cytoplasmic receptor, then localizes in mitochondria and directs oxidative metabolism

(E) None of the above

66. 1,25-Dihydroxycholecalciferol

67. Thyrotropin-releasing hormone

68. Epinephrine

69. Insulin

70. Luteinizing hormone

71. Cortisol

72. Thyroxine

Questions 73–77

For each hormone that follows, select its appropriate function in breast development and lactation.

(A) Plays a background role in breast development

(B) Stimulates development of alveolar components

(C) Stimulates growth of ductal system

(D) Stimulates milk let-down

(E) None of the above

73. Progesterone

74. Estradiol

75. Prolactin

76. Oxytocin

77. Insulin

Questions 78–80

For each situation described below, select the lettered curve on the graph that best represents the blood glucose pattern of the animal in question.

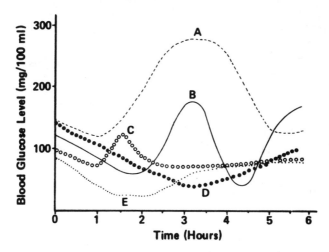

78. A normal dog receives an intravenous injection of pure crystalline insulin without glucose at time zero

79. An alloxan-treated diabetic dog goes without food for 12 h and is given a glucose meal at time 1 h

80. A normal dog goes without food for 12 h and is given glucose at time 1 h

Questions 81–85

For each of the hormones listed below, select the pancreatic islet cell by which it is secreted.

(A) A (α) cell
(B) B (β) cell
(C) D (δ) cell
(D) F cell
(E) None of the above

81. Somatostatin

82. Secretin

83. Insulin

84. Glucagon

85. Pancreatic polypeptide

Metabolism and Endocrinology

Answers

1. The answer is D. *(Berne, 2/e. p 682. Ganong, 15/e. pp 32, 329.)* Paracrine communication is one of three general mechanisms of intercellular communication mediated by chemical messengers. In the paracrine mechanism, chemical messengers produced in response to specific stimuli are released into the extracellular fluid and diffuse locally to influence nearby target cells. The two other mechanisms mediated by chemical messengers are neural communication, in which neurotransmitters released from neurons at synaptic clefts interact in a very confined space with a postsynaptic receptor, and endocrine communication, in which hormones are transmitted via the blood to specific receptors in target tissues. Paracrine communication has been detected in various parts of the central nervous system and gastrointestinal tract, and in the pancreatic islets where somatostatin produced by the D (δ) cells acts locally on the B (β) cells to inhibit insulin secretion.

2. The answer is D. *(West, 12/e. pp 782–785.)* The interaction of a peptide hormone with its receptor is an example of allosteric regulation, a process in which binding of an effector molecule (hormone) to one site on a protein (receptor) alters the conformation of another site on that protein (activity site). Binding of a peptide hormone to its membrane receptor results in coupling between the hormone-binding site and a second active site, which may affect a transport protein or an enzyme, e.g., adenyl cyclase. The binding interactions may involve hydrophobic interactions, hydrogen bonding, or salt bridges but do not involve formation of covalent linkages. Formation of covalent hormone-receptor linkages would make it more difficult to terminate a biologic response once the conditions eliciting it were removed.

3. The answer is A. *(Guyton, 8/e. pp 827–828.)* It is thought that the secretion of antidiuretic hormone (ADH)—also called *arginine vasopressin (AVP)*—and oxytocin by the neurohypophysis is regulated in the hypothalamic supraoptic and paraventricular nuclei, respectively. This hypothalamic control of secretion of pituitary hormone (inhibitory as well as releasing) the case of the neurohypophysis is by direct neural connection, and in case of the adenohypophysis by humoral factors conveyed by a microcirculation known as the *hypothalamic-hypophyseal portal system.*

4. The answer is B. *(Ganong, 15/e. p 329.)* Pancreatic polypeptide is synthesized and secreted by the F cells of the pancreatic islets in response to both vagal and beta-adrenergic stimulation. Its secretion is also increased by protein ingestion, exercise, and acute hypoglycemia. The physiologic role of pancreatic polypeptide has not yet been established, though it does reduce pancreatic enzyme secretion following duodenal perfusion of glucose, amino acids, or oleic acid and may oppose the actions of cholecystokinin.

5. The answer is C. *(Ganong, 15/e. pp 334–335. West, 12/e. p 828.)* During fetal life, the adrenal cortex consists of a thin subcapsular rim, which eventually gives rise to the adult cortex, and a thick inner fetal cortex, which constitutes 80 percent of the gland. This zone undergoes rapid involution after birth. Because it lacks 3β-hydroxysteroid dehydrogenase, the enzyme that converts pregnenolone to progesterone (the initial step in both glucocorticoid and mineralocorticoid synthesis), the fetal cortex synthesizes primarily dehydroepiandrosterone. This steroid is released as its sulfate and is metabolized further to estrogen and androgen by the placenta.

6. The answer is E. *(Berne, 2/e. pp 942–946.)* Thyroid hormone affects all aspects of metabolism; it increases calorigenesis in every tissue in the body. The hormone stimulates protein synthesis, which may be directly responsible for a portion of its calorigenic effect. Thyroid hormone affects both synthesis and degradation of lipids; the net effect is a decrease in lipid stores. By increasing the mechanisms by which cholesterol is eliminated from the body, thyroid hormone decreases plasma cholesterol levels. Because of its stimulatory effect on metabolic processes, thyroid hormone increases the demand for coenzymes and vitamins.

7. The answer is B. *(Guyton, 8/e. pp 746, 857–858.)* Glucose will not diffuse through a cell membrane against a concentration gradient; in many cells diffusion is facilitated in the presence of insulin. Such transport is enhanced, for example, in skeletal, cardiac, some smooth muscle, and adipose tissue. Insulin does not enhance glucose transport into brain cells, through intestinal mucosa, or through tubular epithelium of the kidney.

8. The answer is B. *(Ganong, 15/e. p 273.)* At rest, the caloric needs of the body are met primarily by mitochondrial oxidation of free fatty acids from adipose tissue. Glucose is used primarily by the brain and erythrocytes. During prolonged exercise, skeletal muscle becomes relatively anaerobic when compared with its resting state and relies heavily upon glycolysis for ATP production. The increase in glucose required is met primarily by glycogenolysis and gluconeogenesis in the liver. Gluconeogenesis does not occur in skeletal muscle. Thus, long-distance runners "carbohydrate load" before a race to increase hepatic glycogen stores. Intestinal uptake of glucose is influenced primarily by dietary intake, which would not ordinarily increase during exercise.

9. The answer is D. *(Ganong, 15/e. pp 400–401. West, 12/e. p 874.)* Spermatozoa within the seminiferous tubules are nonmotile and are carried to the epididymis by movement of fluid secreted by the Sertoli cells. While further maturation occurs in the epididymis, ejaculated sperm are still not capable of fertilization. The final steps in sperm maturation, which result in increased motility and acquisition of the capacity to fertilize an egg, occur in the female genital tract and are referred to as *capacitation*. The precise sequence of events has not been fully elucidated but involves release of hydrolytic enzymes from the acrosome, a structure within the sperm head. These hydrolytic enzymes assist in the dispersal of the layer of granulosa cells surrounding the egg and permit the sperm to make contact with microvilli on the plasma membrane of the egg.

10. The answer is A. *(Guyton, 8/e. p 852.)* Removal of the adrenal glands produces the clinical picture known as Addison's disease, a disorder associated with deprivation of adrenocortical hormones. Thus, a lack of glucocorticoids diminishes the body's ability to synthesize glucose by gluconeogenesis. Severe mineralocorticoid deprivation produces grave fluid and electrolyte disturbances as an ultimate consequence of impaired sodium reabsorption, excessive potassium plasma levels, and acidosis.

11. The answer is B. *(Ganong, 15/e. pp 675–676, 679–680.)* Aldosterone acts upon epithelial cells of the nephrons, sweat glands, salivary glands, and the gastrointestinal tract to promote the conservation of sodium and the excretion of potassium. As a consequence of sodium retention, there is a modest expansion of extracellular fluid volume and thus an increase in body weight. With expansion of extracellular volume, blood pressure also increases.

12. The answer is D. *(Ganong, 15/e. p 351.)* Cortisol is the only hormone that has a diurnal variation, as shown in the graph accompanying the question. Plasma cortisol levels rise sharply during sleep, peaking soon after awakening, and sinking to a low level approximately 12 h later. This pattern is intimately related to the secretory rhythm of ACTH, which governs—and in turn is partly governed by—plasma concentration of cortisol.

13. The answer is C. *(Guyton, 8/e. pp 899–903.)* Ovulation takes place just after the peak of the luteinizing hormone (LH) and estrogen curves, which occurs on approximately the fourteenth day of the menstrual cycle. Although FSH is primarily responsible for follicular maturation within the ovary, LH is necessary for final follicular maturation; without it, ovulation cannot take place. Both estrogen, following a sharp preovulatory rise in plasma concentration, and progesterone are secreted in abundance by the postovulatory corpus luteum.

14. The answer is B. *(Guyton, 8/e. pp 831–833.)* The thyroid gland has a specialized active transport system that very efficiently traps iodide from circulating blood and can accumulate iodide against a large concentration gradient. Within the thyroid, the iodide rapidly undergoes organification by which it is oxidized and covalently linked to tyrosine residues in thyroglobulin. Thus, it is in thyroglobulin that iodide is principally stored within the thyroid gland. The iodinated tyrosine residues gradually become coupled to form thyroxine, the major secretion product of the thyroid.

15. The answer is D. *(Guyton 8/e. pp 899–903.)* There is a marked increase in progesterone secretion following ovulation. Almost all the progesterone secreted in nonpregnant women is secreted by the corpus luteum. Secretion of both progesterone and estrogen is controlled by luteinizing hormone (LH) released by the adenohypophysis, and LH release itself is under the direction of a hypothalamic releasing factor.

16. The answer is B. *(Guyton, 8/e. pp 831–833.)* Thyroxine is the main thyroid hormone entering the circulation and constitutes approximately 95 percent of active plasma thyroid hormone; the percentage remaining is almost entirely triiodothyronine, which, although more potent than thyroxine, has a more transient presence. Thyroglobulin is the principal storage form of thyroid hormone within the gland and very little is released into the blood. Thyrotropin (TSH) and long-acting thyroid stimulator (LATS) both stimulate thyroid hormone production and growth of the thyroid gland.

17. The answer is E. *(Guyton, 8/e. p 833.)* Circulating thyroxine can be bound to albumin, thyroxine-binding prealbumin (TBPA), or thyroxine-binding globulin (TBG). Most thyroxine is bound, and despite the large available pool of albumin, most of it is bound to TBG. This reflects the relatively greater affinity of TBG for thyroxine. Only the free unbound form of thyroxine is physiologically active.

18. The answer is E. *(Ganong, 15/e. pp 367–369.)* An increase of parathyroid hormone (PTH) in the body causes an increase in the level of plasma calcium by mobilizing calcium from bones and by increasing reabsorption of calcium in the kidneys. It also increases intestinal absorption of calcium by increasing formation of 1,25-dihydroxycholecalciferol. PTH causes a decrease in the level of plasma phosphate by decreasing renal proximal tubular reabsorption of phosphate. Despite increased renal reabsorption of calcium, hypercalciuria occurs and kidney stones containing calcium are commonly formed during hyperparathyroidism because the increased amount of calcium filtered exceeds the renal reabsorptive capacity.

19. The answer is D. *(Guyton, 8/e. pp 746, 857–858.)* Insulin increases glucose uptake in skeletal muscle, cardiac muscle, smooth muscle, adipose tissue, leukocytes, and the liver. It does not do so in the brain (except probably in part of the hypothalamus), renal tubules, intestinal mucosa, or red blood cells. In most insulin-sensitive tissues, insulin acts to promote glucose transport by enhancing facilitated diffusion of glucose down a concentration gradient. In the liver, where glucose freely permeates the cell membrane, glucose uptake is increased as a result of its phosphorylation by glucokinase. Formation of glucose-6-phosphate reduces the intracellular concentration of free glucose and maintains the concentration gradient favoring movement of glucose into the cell.

20. The answer is E. *(Guyton, 8/e. pp 746–747, 835.)* Epinephrine and glucagon stimulate glycogenolysis in the liver by means of a mechanism dependent on cyclic adenosine monophosphate. Thyroxine, glucagon, and ACTH (by increasing cortisol secretion) also enhance gluconeogenesis from amino acid precursors. Both of these processes result in hyperglycemia. Aldosterone, a mineralocorticoid involved in sodium regulation, has no direct effect on glucose metabolism.

21. The answer is C. *(Berne, 2/e. pp 1006–1010. Guyton, 8/e. pp 899–902.)* Preparation of primordial ovarian follicles for ovulation is the primary function of follicle-stimulating hormone (FSH). During the initial 10 to 14 days of the menstrual cycle, secretion of FSH stimulates development of the theca and granulosa cells of the follicle and promotes their synthesis of estrogens, including estradiol. When estrogen reaches a certain level, a sudden surge of secretion of FSH and luteinizing hormone (LH) occurs, followed by ovulation. The surge in LH then promotes luteinization of the postovulatory follicle and stimulates the production of progesterone by the resultant corpus luteum. If pregnancy occurs, chorionic gonadotropin (hCG) is secreted by the placenta and replaces the stimulation of production of progesterone by LH.

22. The answer is B. *(Ganong, 15/e. pp 426–429. Guyton, 8/e. pp 211–215.)* Angiotensin II is an octapeptide produced in response to hypovolemia by the combined action of renin, released from the juxtaglomerular apparatus, and angiotensin-converting enzyme in the lung. It has a number of actions, all of which are directed toward increasing arterial pressure. The actions include (1) direct vasoconstriction of peripheral arterioles; (2) stimulation of aldosterone secretion by the adrenal cortex, resulting in increased sodium tubular resorption; and (3) stimulation of the subfornical organ of the diencephalon, which activates neural areas concerned with thirst. The latter two actions, by increasing blood volume, play a role in long-term regulation of blood pressure. Angiotensin II also exerts negative feedback on its own production by inhibiting renin secretion. It does not act directly on renal tubules to influence salt excretion.

23. The answer is E. *(Ganong, 15/e. pp 87, 230, 329, 453. Guyton, 8/e. pp 825–826.)* Somatostatin is a short-lived tetradecapeptide that is secreted at several sites, including the D cells of the pancreatic islets, the hypothalamus, and the vagus nerve. Because its half-life in plasma is only 1 to 3 min owing to rapid degradation, it is believed to exert its effects in close proximity to its site of release. It has been shown to inhibit secretion of a variety of hormones, including growth hormone, gastrin, insulin, and glucagon, and thus has a widespread role in modulating multiple hormonal systems.

24. The answer is C. *(Berne, 2/e. pp 943–947.)* Hypothyroidism is a condition usually characterized by low levels of T_3 and T_4 owing to atrophy of the thyroid gland. In very rare cases there is resistance to the effects of thyroid hormones. A deficiency of thyroid hormones or their effects results in bradycardia, which is due to decreased sympathetic activity, and a decreased metabolic rate with its associated sleepiness, weight gain, and cold intolerance. Excess thyroid hormones increase metabolic rate, which increases heat production, stimulates the appetite, and causes weight loss even in the face of increased intake of food. Heat intolerance is characteristic of hyperthyroidism.

25. The answer is E. *(Guyton, 8/e. pp 907–908.)* In response to estrogen secretion by the ovary, the endometrial lining of the uterus undergoes proliferation of both glandular epithelium and supporting stroma during the first 10 to 14 days of the menstrual cycle. Following ovulation (point A on the graph accompanying the question) the glands begin to secrete mucus and the stroma undergoes pseudodecidual reaction in preparation for potential pregnancy. When ovulation is not followed by implantation of a fertilized ovum, progesterone secretion declines as the corpus luteum involutes, and the endometrial lining is almost completely shed during menses.

26. The answer is D. *(Ganong, 15/e. pp 306–311. Guyton, 8/e. pp 838–840.)* Goiter, or thyroid enlargement, can occur in association with any level of thyroid function. Thyroid growth is controlled primarily by thyroid-stimulating hormone (TSH). Increased levels of TSH could occur with a pituitary adenoma or as a consequence of diminished negative feedback by thyroid hormone on the hypothalamus owing to decreased synthesis of the hormone. A decrease in synthesis of thyroid hormone would accompany iodine deficiency or ingestion of goitrogens, which inhibit iodination reactions in the thyroid. Goitrogens may be found in cabbage or turnips. In Graves' disease, an immunoglobulin that binds to TSH receptors causes an increase in thyroid size. Excessive intake of thyroxine would suppress TSH secretion and not cause thyroid enlargement.

27. The answer is B. *(Ganong, 15/e. pp 403–407. Guyton, 8/e. pp 891–894.)* Testosterone, the major androgenic steroid, is synthesized from cholesterol in the interstitial Leydig cells of the testis in response to luteinizing hormone (LH). It exerts negative feedback on pituitary secretion of LH by inhibiting release of gonadotropin-releasing hormone from the hypothalamus. Testosterone circulates in the serum bound to protein, principally to a beta globulin known as *gonadal steroid-binding globulin*. Reduction of testosterone to the more physiologically active dihydrotestosterone occurs in some target tissues. Testosterone is an intermediate in the biosynthesis of estrogen in both male and female and is inactivated in the liver by oxidation to 17-ketosteroids.

28. The answer is A. *(Guyton, 8/e. pp 919–920.)* Human chorionic gonadotropin (hCG) begins to appear in the maternal blood approximately 6 to 8 days following ovulation, upon implantation of the fertilized ovum in the endometrium. The secretion of hCG is essential to prevent involution of the corpus luteum and to stimulate secretion of progesterone and estrogens, which continues until the placenta becomes large enough to secrete sufficient quantities of those hormones. Following a peak at 7 to 9 weeks, hCG secretion gradually declines to a low level by 20 weeks gestation.

29. The answer is B. *(Guyton, 8/e. pp 524–525, 851.)* Endorphins (α-, β-, γ-endorphins), a group of endogenous opiates recently isolated from brain tissue and the pituitary, are peptides that function as neurotransmitters at many loci within the brain and influence peripheral neural function, especially in the gastrointestinal tract. These substances have morphinelike actions in that they raise the pain threshold. Endorphins are synthesized as part of a larger polypeptide molecule that includes the sequence for ACTH and β-lipotropin, and melanocyte-stimulating hormone (MSH). During periods of stress, the pituitary secretes increased amounts of both ACTH and endorphin.

30. The answer is C. *(West, 12/e. pp 801–802.)* Synthesis and secretion of growth hormone by the anterior pituitary is regulated by a variety of metabolic factors, many of which act to alter the balance between release of growth hormone–releasing hormone (GRH) and somatostatin (SS) from the hypothalamus. Insulin-induced hypoglycemia is a major stimulus for release of growth hormone. Amino acids are also potent stimuli for release of growth hormone, while fatty acids are inhibitory. Deep sleep induces the greatest daily peak in secretion of growth hormone. Thyroxine acts directly on pituitary cells to enhance synthesis of growth hormone and is required for the normal responsiveness of the pituitary and hypothalamus to physiologic stimuli.

31. The answer is A. *(West, 12/e. pp 761–763.)* Most, if not all, of the effects of insulin begin with the binding of insulin to its specific membrane receptor. This binding is associated with autophosphorylation of tyrosine residues in the receptor molecule and exhibits "negative cooperativity"; that is, binding of one molecule of insulin reduces the affinity of the receptor for a second molecule of insulin that would completely saturate its binding sites. Prolonged elevation of plasma insulin levels leads to a reduction in the number of available receptor molecules ("down-regulation") so that the effect of a given dose of insulin is diminished. Insulin-receptor binding is required for initiation of the effects of insulin on the enhanced transport of glucose, amino acids, and potassium into cells.

32. The answer is B. *(Ganong, 15/e. p 287. West, 12/e. pp 744–746.)* Hormone-sensitive lipase is a cytoplasmic enzyme in adipocytes that catalyzes the complete hydrolysis of triglyceride to fatty acids and glycerol. It is activated by a cyclic AMP–dependent protein kinase that phosphorylates the enzyme, converting it to its active form. Since no accumulation of monoglycerides or diglycerides is detected in adipocytes following the action of hormone-sensitive lipase, it is the initial hydrolysis of triglyceride to fatty acid and diglyceride that is the rate-limiting step. Hormone-sensitive lipase is sensitive to several hormones in vitro, but it appears to be regulated in vivo primarily by epinephrine and glucagon, which activate it by increasing cyclic AMP, and insulin, which inhibits it by preventing cyclic AMP–dependent phosphorylation. Cortisol enhances lipolysis indirectly by promoting increased enzyme synthesis.

33. The answer is A. *(Ganong, 15/e. pp 262–264.)* The basal metabolic rate (BMR) is the metabolic rate measured at rest 12 to 14 h after a meal. It is influenced by a number of factors and correlates well with body surface area. Increases in epinephrine secretion, which occur in an anxious person even at rest, increase metabolic rate. Environmental temperature also influences BMR. At low temperatures (e.g., 20°C) heat-conserving mechanisms are activated and BMR rises. At elevated environmental temperatures (e.g., 35 to 40°C) when body temperature also rises slightly, BMR again rises. BMR is high in children and decreases with advancing age.

34. The answer is E. *(West, 12/e. pp 746–747.)* The uptake of triglycerides into adipose tissue and other tissues from plasma lipoproteins requires hydrolysis of triglyceride to fatty acids and glycerol by an enzyme bound to the endothelial surface, lipoprotein lipase. The activity of this enzyme varies in reciprocal fashion with that of cytoplasmic hormone-sensitive lipase; e.g., its activity is enhanced by insulin and glucose and decreased by catecholamines. Lipoprotein lipase is present in nearly every tissue and acts at the capillary surface as it does in adipose tissue. Receptor-mediated endocytosis is important in the turnover of the protein portion of plasma lipoproteins.

35. The answer is D. *(Berne, 2/e. pp 990–997. West, 12/e. pp 851–853, 858–859.)* Spermatogenesis occurs within the seminiferous tubules of the testis and requires secretion of both FSH and LH. FSH acts directly on the seminiferous tubules while the effects of LH are thought to be due to its stimulation of secretion of testosterone by the Leydig cells. Spermatogonia are the stem cells, which divide several times by mitosis to produce more stem cells and type B spermatogonia. The type B spermatogonia give rise to primary spermatocytes, which undergo meiosis. Normally, 100 to 200 million sperm are produced per day. Complete maturation of spermatozoa within the seminiferous tubules requires approximately 70 days in man.

36. The answer is C. *(West, 12/e. pp 851, 856, 858–859.)* The Sertoli cells rest on a basal lamina and form a layer around the periphery of the seminiferous tubules. They are attached to each other by specialized junctional complexes that limit the movement of fluid and solute molecules from the interstitial space and blood to the tubular lumen and thus form a blood-testis barrier that provides an immunologically privileged environment for sperm maturation. Sertoli cells are intimately associated with developing spermatozoa and play a major role in germ-cell maturation. They secrete a variety of serum proteins and an androgen-binding protein into the tubular fluid in response to FSH and testosterone stimulation. Testosterone is synthesized and secreted by the interstitial Leydig cells. Estrogen is produced in small amounts by the Sertoli cells before puberty.

37. The answer is D. *(Ganong, 15/e. pp 421–422. West, 12/e. pp 874–876.)* Fertilization and early cleavage of the zygote occur in the fallopian tube in the human female. After approximately 3 days, the zygote enters the uterine cavity, where it undergoes additional divisions over a period of 3 to 4 days to form a morula of approximately 60 cells that is transformed into a blastocyst consisting of the yolk sac and embryo. Enzymatic digestion of the zona pellucida and infiltration of the endometrium by the syncytiotrophoblast, which forms the outer layer of the blastocyst, result in implantation of the blastocyst within the endometrium, where it erodes into maternal vessels. During these early stages of embryogenesis, the endometrium is primed by progesterone secreted by the corpus luteum in the ovary in response to pituitary gonadotropin secretion. After 10 to 15 days, placental gonadotropins maintain the corpus luteum until placental synthesis of progesterone is established at 6 to 8 weeks of gestation.

38. The answer is B. *(West, 12/e. pp 859–861.)* Genital duct differentiation is completed during the third month of fetal life. In males, testosterone secreted by the testicular Leydig cells promotes differentiation of the wolffian duct system, which gives rise to the epididymis, vas deferens, seminal vesicles, and ejaculatory duct. A glycoprotein (müllerian duct inhibitory, or regression, factor), which is secreted by Sertoli cells in the fetal seminiferous tubules, stimulates simultaneous regression of the müllerian duct system. Persons with testicular feminization lack androgen receptors and thus do not undergo androgen-dependent differentiation of the wolffian system or external genitalia. Because they do synthesize müllerian regression factor, their müllerian duct systems regress, so that they are genetic males but have female external genitalia and lack a uterus and fallopian tubes.

39. The answer is D. *(Ganong, 15/e. p 343.)* Inappropriate virilization manifested by frontal balding and increased facial hair in a female could be a result of excessive amounts of exogenous or endogenous androgens. Small amounts of androgens are normally produced in the female by the adrenal glands and ovaries. Thus, tumors of either the adrenal or ovary might be associated with virilization. Deficiency of 11β-hydroxylase, by leading to hypersecretion of 11-deoxycortisol and 11-deoxycorticosterone, a weak mineralocorticoid, results in a diversion of steroid precursors to androgen-synthesizing pathways. A patient thus affected would manifest both virilization and hypertension.

40. The answer is D. *(Ganong, 15/e. pp 300–301.)* Less than 0.2 percent of plasma triiodothyronine and thyroxine circulate as the free molecule. The three major proteins that bind these hormones in the blood are (1) thyroxine-binding globulin (TBG), (2) thyroxine-binding prealbumin (TBPA), and (3) albumin. Of the three, albumin has the greatest capacity for hormone binding, but its affinity for thyroid hormone is relatively low. Consequently, most of the triiodothyronine and thyroxine circulate bound to TBG and TBPA. Only the free form of the hormone is physiologically active. Thyroglobulin is the form in which the thyroid hormones are stored within the thyroid.

41. The answer is B. *(Guyton, 8/e. pp 831–835.)* Thyroglobulin, the storage form of thyroid hormones, is stored extracellularly in follicles lined by thyroid epithelium. Only about 0.02 percent of the thyroxine and about 0.2 percent of the triiodothyronine are normally present in plasma in the free form; the rest is bound to thyroxine-binding globulin, thyroxine-binding prealbumin, and albumin. Following injection of thyroxine into a human, the effect on the metabolic rate is not noticeable for 2 to 3 days; then the rate begins to increase progressively and reaches a maximum in 10 to 12 days. Some of the activity persists for up to 2 months. The principal effect of the thyroid hormones is an increase in the metabolic rate of most tissues in the body, with a few exceptions such as brain, retina, testes, spleen, and lungs.

42. The answer is C. *(Guyton, 8/e. pp 361–362.)* Iron is transported in the blood plasma bound to the beta globulin transferrin. Excess iron is stored in all cells, but especially in liver cells, combined with the protein apoferritin; the storage complex of iron plus protein is called *ferritin*. The rate of iron absorption is extremely slow, with a maximal rate of only a few milligrams per day. Iron absorption is an active process. Because iron is absorbed mainly in the ferrous rather than ferric form, ferrous iron compounds are more effective in treating iron deficiency than are ferric compounds.

43. The answer is B. *(Ganong, 15/e. pp 432–434.)* Melatonin is synthesized in the pineal gland from the amino acid tryptophan. Synthesis and secretion of melatonin are increased in the dark via input from norepinephrine secreted by postganglionic sympathetic neurons. Pinealomas (tumors of the pineal gland) that destroy the pineal gland, reduce secretion of melatonin, and cause hypothalamic damage may cause precocious puberty by removing the inhibitory effect of melatonin on the pituitary response to gonadotropin-releasing hormone. Melatonin causes amphibian skin to become lighter in color but has no role in the regulation of skin color in humans.

44. The answer is E. *(Ganong, 15/e. pp 312–313.)* The islets of Langerhans, which constitute 1 to 2 percent of the weight of the pancreas, contain at least four types of cells: A (α), B (β), D (δ), and F cells. The A cells secrete glucagon, the B cells secrete insulin, the D cells secrete somatostatin, and the F cells secrete pancreatic polypeptide. There are more islets in the tail than in the head or body of the pancreas, and each islet has a copious blood supply.

45. The answer is E. *(Guyton, 8/e. pp 855–860.)* α-Glycerophosphate is produced in the course of normal use of glucose. In the absence of adequate quantities of α-glycerophosphate—a normal acceptor of free fatty acids in triglyceride synthesis—lipolysis will be the predominant process in adipose tissue. As a result, fatty acids will be released into the blood. The prevailing insulin level is decisive in the selection of substrate by a tissue for the production of energy. Insulin promotes use of carbohydrate, and a lack of the hormone causes use of fat mainly to the exclusion of uptake and use of glucose, except by brain tissue. Indirect depression of use of glucose by excess fatty acids is a result, and not a contributing cause, of increased use of fat.

46. The answer is D. *(Ganong, 15/e. pp 324–326.)* Blood glucose levels affect the pancreatic islets directly and constitute the major control mechanism of insulin secretion; adequate quantities of Ca^{2+} and K^+ are also required for normal secretion. 2-Deoxyglucose, a nonmetabolized analogue of glucose, inhibits insulin secretion, as does somatostatin, a polypeptide present in the D (δ) cells of the pancreatic islets (and in several other tissues). Thiazide diuretics, not an osmotic diuretic such as the inert sugar mannitol, inhibit insulin secretion in some patients.

47. The answer is D. *(Ganong, 15/e. pp 367–369.)* The main function of the parathyroid gland is to maintain a constant ionized calcium level in the extracellular fluid. To do this, parathyroid hormone stimulates increased plasma calcium levels, chiefly by mobilizing calcium from bones. Although parathyroid hormone can also increase renal tubular reabsorption of calcium and intestinal absorption of calcium, these effects depend on adequate dietary ingestion of calcium and thus occur more slowly.

48. The answer is A. *(Ganong, 15/e. pp 368–371.)* Parathyroid hormone is essential for maintaining normal plasma calcium and phosphate concentrations. Parathyroid hormone is released in response to low plasma calcium concentrations and acts to increase phosphate excretion and calcium reabsorption. If parathyroid hormone concentrations rise above normal levels, plasma calcium concentrations will increase and plasma concentrations of phosphate will decrease. Calcitonin is released by the thyroid gland when plasma concentrations of calcium increase. Thus the increase in calcium associated with hyperparathyroidism will cause an increase in the secretion of calcitonin. Sodium and potassium levels are not affected by a decrease in parathyroid hormone levels.

49. The answer is B. *(Berne, 2/e. pp 915–919.)* Human growth hormone (GH) is a peptide that is synthesized and released from the anterior pituitary. Its release is stimulated by growth hormone–releasing hormone (GHRH) and inhibited by somatostatin. Both of these peptides are synthesized and released by the hypothalamus and their releases are regulated by multiple feedback loops. GH has the direct effect on adipose tissue of decreasing glucose uptake and increasing lipolysis. It also acts to increase the production and release of somatomedins from the liver. These peptides have a multitude of effects on the body and promote growth of organs, bones, and lean body mass.

50. The answer is D. *(Berne, 2/e. pp 1011–1012, 1016–1018.)* The plasma level of progesterone is low during the menses and remains low until just prior to ovulation. It rises substantially after ovulation owing to secretion by the corpus luteum. If fertilization occurs, the corpus luteum continues to secrete progesterone until the placenta develops and begins to produce large amounts of the hormone. The plasma level of progesterone rises steadily throughout pregnancy after the placenta takes over production at about 12 weeks of gestation.

51. The answer is C. *(Ganong, 15/e. p 349. Guyton, 8/e. pp 848–849.)* The anti-inflammatory effects of exogenous cortisol are due to its ability to decrease capillary membrane permeability and probably also to its ability to stabilize lysosomal membranes and decrease the formation of bradykinin. Glucocorticoids inhibit the enzyme phospholipase A_2. This decreases the release of arachidonic acid and the variety of substances produced from it, such as leukotrienes, prostaglandins, thromboxanes, and prostacyclin. Cortisol owes its fever-reducing action to the hormone's ability to decrease the release of pyrogen (interleukin 1) from granulocytes. However, only in massive doses will the hormone achieve the effects described. Endogenous cortisol does not exert significant anti-inflammatory action.

52. The answer is E. *(Ganong, 15/e. pp 411–416.)* Estrogens can stimulate growth of ovarian follicles even in hypophysectomized women. Estrogens also stimulate growth of the glandular epithelium of the endometrium, the smooth muscle of the uterus, and the uterine vascular system. The epithelium of the vagina is so sensitive to estrogen action that vaginal smear examination is used for a bioassay of the hormone. Estrogens cause the mucus secreted by the cervix to become thinner and more alkaline and to exhibit a fernlike pattern upon drying. Growth of the *glandular* elements of the breast is stimulated by progesterone; growth of the *ductal* elements is stimulated by estrogen.

53. The answer is D. *(Guyton, 8/e. pp 822–824.)* Growth hormone exerts a wide variety of effects on body metabolism, including increased protein synthesis, decreased use of carbohydrate, and increased use of fat. The net effect of the hormone's action is the accumulation of protein and conservation of carbohydrate at the expense of fat stores. In addition to those effects, growth hormone promotes growth by stimulating synthesis of cartilage and bone via the actions of somatomedin C (insulin-like growth factor 1 [IGF-1]).

54. The answer is C. *(Ganong, 15/e. pp 326–327. Guyton, 8/e. pp 862–863.)* The primary action of glucagon is to increase blood glucose concentration, which it accomplishes by promoting gluconeogenesis and glycogenolysis in the liver but not in muscle. These effects are mediated by cyclic AMP, which is produced by hepatic adenyl cyclase following interaction of glucagon with its plasma membrane receptor. Interaction of glucagon with different hepatic plasma membrane receptors activates phospholipase C, which results in a rise in concentration of intracellular Ca^{2+}, which further stimulates glycogenolysis. Although glucagon opposes the action of insulin, it does not directly affect insulin secretion.

55. The answer is D. *(Ganong, 15/e. p 369.)* The major action of parathyroid hormone is to increase plasma calcium concentration by mobilization of calcium from bones, increasing absorption of calcium by the intestine, and decreasing the secretion of calcium by the kidney. When a person is unable to secrete a normal amount of parathyroid hormone, calcium levels fall, which leads to tetany, a condition in which the excitability of nerves and muscles increases. The increase in excitability results from a lowering of the voltage at which an action potential can be elicited. Threshold can be reduced so low that tapping a muscle can cause it to contract.

56. The answer is C. *(Ganong, 15/e. pp 339–342.)* Cholesterol is the precursor for biosynthesis of all adrenal steroids. The rate-limiting step in their biosynthesis is conversion of cholesterol to pregnenolone by stepwise hydroxylation. From that point, divergent pathways result in synthesis of glucocorticoids (cortisol and corticosterone), mineralocorticoids (aldosterone), and small amounts of estrogen (estradiol) and androgen (testosterone). Dexamethasone is a synthetic steroid with potent glucocorticoid activity.

57. The answer is A. *(Ganong, 15/e. pp 300, 305–306.)* Thyroid-stimulating hormone (TSH) increases all metabolic activities of thyroid glandular cells, including thyroglobulin proteolysis and iodide pumping, and it has a trophic influence on the thyroid, which results in an increase in the number and size of thyroid epithelial cells. Its secretion from the anterior pituitary is modulated by thyrotropin-releasing hormone, which is released from the hypothalamus, as well as by somatostatin, which has an inhibitory effect on TSH secretion. The effects of TSH on the thyroid are mediated by cyclic AMP, which is formed by adenyl cyclase following TSH receptor interaction. Most of the circulating thyroid hormone is bound to plasma proteins (albumin, globulin, and thyroxine-binding protein). TSH has no effect on the concentration of thyroxine-binding protein.

58. The answer is A. *(Ganong, 15/e. pp 421–423.)* During early pregnancy, human chorionic gonadotropin (hCG) secretion increases steadily, reaching a peak at 8 to 9 weeks following implantation of the fertilized ovum. Estriol and pregnanediol—estrogen and progesterone metabolites—are excreted in the urine. Their excretion and that of human chorionic somatomammotropin (hCS), a peptide hormone similar to human growth hormone, increase steadily and peak just before parturition. Oxytocin is important in the development of uterine contractions during labor and is secreted in the greatest amounts only at parturition, when uterine sensitivity to the hormone is maximal.

59. The answer is D. *(Ganong, 15/e. pp 403–404, 414.)* Testosterone synthesis begins with the conversion of cholesterol to pregnenolone by stepwise hydroxylation. Pregnenolone is then converted to dehydroepiandrosterone, which can then undergo conversion to androstenedione and then to testosterone, a 17-hydroxysteroid. Estrogens can be formed from testosterone by stepwise reduction of the 3-keto group and ring aromatization. Those steps are irreversible; hence estrogen is not a precursor for testosterone.

60. The answer is C. *(Ganong, 15/e. pp 326–328.)* Glucagon is a peptide hormone secreted by the A (α) cells of the pancreatic islets. It acts to raise the blood glucose level. It also binds to receptors on liver cells and causes an increase in the cytosolic level of cyclic AMP. This stimulates the enzyme phosphorylase to break down glycogen into glucose. Glucagon does not stimulate glycogenolysis in muscle. It does stimulate the liver to make glucose from amino acids (gluconeogenesis) and increases lipolysis in adipose tissue. The fatty acids produced can then be taken up by the liver and be used to produce ketone bodies.

61. The answer is A. *(Ganong, 15/e. pp 313–315. Guyton, 8/e. pp 855–856.)* Proinsulin, a single-chain polypeptide, is a precursor of insulin. The insulin molecule is composed of two polypeptide chains, which are linked via disulfide bonds. In proinsulin these two chains are linked by an intervening peptide sequence termed *C (connecting) peptide*. Cleavage of proinsulin to insulin and C peptide takes place in the Golgi complex so that equimolar amounts of insulin and C peptide are secreted by the β cell. Proinsulin shows some immunologic cross-reactivity with insulin but is much less biologically active.

62. The answer is D. *(Ganong, 15/e. pp 315–318.)* One of insulin's major effects is the stimulation of the Na-K pump, which increases potassium entry into cells. Insulin given along with glucose, to prevent hypoglycemia, is often used as a treatment for hyperkalemia. Insulin's major effect on metabolism is the synthesis of proteins and lipids and the storage of glucose as glycogen. Insulin stimulates the uptake of amino acids and glucose by most cells of the body and decreases the rate of gluconeogenesis. Insulin has no effect on urine formation, but in diabetes, when glucose levels increase to a level at which the kidney can no longer reabsorb the filtered glucose, glucose acts as an osmotic diuretic and increases the formation of urine.

63. The answer is A. *(Ganong, 15/e. pp 350–353.)* The secretion of ACTH occurs in several irregular bursts during the day; the peak occurs early in the morning prior to awakening and thus is not due to the stress of arising. This circadian rhythm—maximum secretion in early morning, minimum in the evening—is regulated by the hypothalamus through the secretion of corticotropin-releasing hormone (CRH) into the hypothalamic-hypophyseal portal capillary system. In addition to the basal rhythm, physical or mental stress will lead to increased ACTH secretion within minutes. ACTH is also regulated as a result of feedback inhibition by the hormones whose synthesis it stimulates, e.g., glucocorticoids. Aldosterone is a mineralocorticoid and not controlled by ACTH. Epinephrine does not appear to have any effect on ACTH secretion.

64. The answer is D. *(Ganong, 15/e. pp 296–302.)* Thyroxine (T_4) is the principal secretory product of the thyroid. Conversion of T_4 to triiodothyronine (T_3) occurs at a variety of extrathyroidal sites and precedes many of the physiologic actions of thyroid hormones, which suggests that the conversion may be necessary for hormone action. This hypothesis is confirmed by the observation that T_3 is more potent than T_4 in many systems. Decreased conversion of T_4 to T_3 occurs in altered physiologic states characterized by acute or chronic caloric deprivation, including starvation, trauma, and diabetes.

65. The answer is E. *(Ganong, 15/e. pp 406–408. Guyton, 8/e. pp 896–897.)* Because gonadotropin secretion from the anterior pituitary gland is regulated by the secretion of gonadotropin-releasing hormone from the hypothalamus, it is not surprising that lesions in either of those sites would curtail gonadotropin production and result in hypogonadism. The pineal gland, located in the roof of the third ventricle, has been ascribed a variety of functions; it was originally described by Descartes as the seat of the soul. In animals, its activation by external light influences gonadotropin secretion. Although the function of the pineal gland in humans is unclear, pineal tumors are often associated with altered gonadotropin secretion. The testes are the major site of testosterone production. Testosterone is responsible for promoting and maintaining male secondary sex characteristics and sperm production.

66–72. The answers are: 66-B, 67-A, 68-A, 69-C, 70-A, 71-B, 72-B. *(Berne, 2/e. pp 825–831.)* Hormones can be divided into two major groups on the basis of their mechanisms of action and biochemical properties: (1) the lipid-soluble hormones, which include adrenal (cortisol) and gonadal steroids, the iodothyronines (thyroxine), and vitamin D (cholecalciferol), and (2) the water-soluble peptide (LH, thyrotropin-releasing hormone, insulin) and catecholamine (epinephrine) hormones.

The lipid-soluble hormones, because of their limited water solubility, are transported in the plasma bound to proteins. They are able to penetrate the plasma membrane readily and interact with specific cytoplasmic receptors that solubilize them and transport them to the nucleus. Within the nucleus, the hormones act on specific receptors to stimulate the production of specific messenger RNA, which then directs the synthesis of specific protein products. These effects occur over a period of hours so that the physiologic response follows an initial lag period after hormone exposure. The mechanism by which these hormones influence nuclear function is still unclear. Characterization of cytoplasmic and nuclear receptors has indicated that they are proteins that bind their ligands with high specificity. The proteins have been partially purified and are characterized primarily by their ultracentrifugal sedimentation behavior and their affinity for their ligand.

The peptide and catecholamine hormones are water-soluble and circulate unbound in the plasma and extracellular fluid. These hormones bind to cell surface receptors in their target tissues and do not require penetration of the plasma membrane for their actions. In some cases, hormone-receptor complexes are internalized and degraded via lysosomal hydrolysis. Following interaction with their receptors, these hormones stimulate production of intracellular mediators, which function as "second messengers" for the "first messenger" (hormone). For many peptide and catecholamine hormones the intracellular messenger is a cyclic nucleotide, i.e., cyclic $3',5'$-adenosine monophosphate (cAMP) or cyclic $3',5'$-guanosine monophosphate (cGMP). The cyclic nucleotides are synthesized by membrane-bound nucleotide cyclases, which are coupled to hormone receptors by several intervening protein interactions. The cyclic nucleotides exert a variety of effects depending on the target tissue. The specificity of the hormone response is mediated by the hormone receptor and the metabolic capabilities of the target cell. Thus, although the two hormones luteinizing hormone and thyrotropin-releasing hormone both activate adenyl cyclase, they do so only in the target tissues that possess their receptors. One well-characterized mechanism of action of cyclic nucleotides is the activation of protein kinases to catalyze the phosphorylation of various protein substrates. Again, the specificity of the response depends on the properties of the target cell and the protein substrates available for phosphorylation. An example of this mechanism is the activation of phosphorylase in response to epinephrine in the liver.

A notable exception to the cyclic nucleotide second messenger mechanism is insulin, a polypeptide hormone that acts on a variety of target cells to alter carbohydrate, lipid, and protein metabolism. Although it is clear that insulin exerts its actions by binding to a plasma membrane receptor, the nature of its second messenger is still the subject of intense investigation.

It has been shown that another level of regulation characterizing hormone-sensitive systems involves the control of the number and affinity of receptors in the target cell membrane. Thus, changes in receptor number and density may be responsible for some of the diseases previously thought to result from an apparent deficiency in hormone secretion.

73–77. The answers are: 73-B, 74-C, 75-B, 76-D, 77-A. *(Ganong, 15/e. pp 415, 423–425. Guyton, 8/e. pp 925–927.)* Breast development depends on the coordinated action of numerous hormones including prolactin, progesterone, estrogen, insulin, growth hormone, thyroid hormone, and glucocorticoids. The precise role of individual hormones is difficult to establish because each hormone may influence the secretion of others. In general, estrogens promote duct growth and progesterone and prolactin are essential for lobular development. The contributions of insulin, glucocorticoids, growth hormone, and thyroid hormone are not clear. Their presence appears to be necessary for breast development although some degree of breast function may occur in the presence of isolated deficiencies. Mineralocorticoids do not appear to be involved in breast development.

The primary hormone governing breast development and function is prolactin, which is secreted by the anterior pituitary. Its presence is required in order for estrogen and progesterone to influence breast development. Plasma prolactin levels are elevated during pregnancy as the breast is prepared for lactation. Following delivery, prolactin levels gradually decline. Suckling of the breast by the nursing infant produces a burst of prolactin secretion that subsides once feeding is completed. Such bursts of prolactin secretion are required for maintenance of the breast in an actively lactating state.

Oxytocin is a posterior pituitary peptide that promotes contraction of the myoepithelial cells surrounding breast ducts and causes expulsion of milk from lobular alveoli. Secretion of oxytocin is promoted by tactile stimulation of the breast by the nursing infant. It can also be elicited by psychic factors alone, such as the anticipation of nursing brought on by hearing the cry of the hungry infant. This anticipatory secretion of oxytocin may be experienced by the mother as a sensation of milk let-down in which milk appears at the nipple and may be forcibly ejected. Prolactin secretion is not subject to anticipatory psychic stimuli.

Estrogens, which play a complex role in mammary development, require the presence of growth hormone as well as prolactin. While promoting ductal development, estrogens actually inhibit lactation. The abrupt withdrawal of estrogen at parturition is one of the stimuli responsible for the onset of lactation. Nuclear and cytoplasmic estrogen receptors have been demonstrated in mammary tissue and have been used clinically to attempt to define the biologic potential for breast malignancy.

Progesterone receptors are also present in breast tissue. Progesterone acts synergistically with prolactin to promote lobular development.

78–80. The answers are: 78-E, 79-A, 80-C. *(Berne, 2/e. pp 855–856, 860–863, 871–872. Ganong, 15/e. pp 331–333.)* Blood glucose levels are maintained by the actions of insulin and a variety of hormones that antagonize insulin action. Following oral intake of glucose, blood levels of glucose rise as glucose is absorbed from the gut (curve C in the graph accompanying the question). This rise in blood glucose level is not sustained because insulin secretion is stimulated. Insulin promotes glucose uptake into muscle and adipose tissue and thus reduces blood glucose concentration.

Administration of insulin without glucose results in hypoglycemia (curve E), a situation that occurs in diabetes mellitus when insulin injections are continued in the absence of adequate oral intake of glucose and that can lead to insulin shock. Severe depression of the brain—an organ that depends almost exclusively on glucose—may result from marked hypoglycemia and is a life-threatening situation that can be reversed by prompt infusion of glucose.

Alloxan is a β-cell antagonist that blocks glucose-stimulated insulin release and acts as a β-cell toxin. Thus, an alloxan-treated animal would manifest glucose tolerance similar to that of an insulin-deficient diabetic. Blood glucose levels would rise to very high levels because of limited glucose uptake in peripheral tissues in the absence of insulin (curve A).

81–85. The answers are: 81-C, 82-E, 83-B, 84-A, 85-D. *(West, 12/e. pp 754–755, 759.)* The endocrine pancreas consists of several hundred thousand nests of cells called islets of Langerhans. Most of these islets are located in the tail and body of the pancreas. The islets are entirely independent of the pancreatic ductal system and exocrine pancreas and secrete their hormones directly into the blood. The reason for the intimate physical relationship between endocrine and exocrine organs is unknown. In some lower species, they are anatomically separate.

The islets consist of at least four cell types, which can be distinguished by electron microscopy because their secretory granules are morphologically different. The cells can also be distinguished with the light microscope by immunohistochemical techniques. In these techniques, specific antibodies (e.g., rabbit anti-insulin) to the hormones are applied to microscopic sections of tissue (e.g., human pancreas), and their binding sites in the tissue are identified by applying a second antibody (e.g., goat antirabbit immunoglobulin) that is covalently linked to a fluorescent dye or enzyme that can be directly visualized following a nonspecific chemical reaction.

Morphological studies using these techniques have shown that the cells of the islets are not randomly distributed. The B (β) cells, which secrete insulin, are the most abundant and make up the central portion of the islets. These cells are recognized with the electron microscope by the β granules, which are membrane-bound organelles containing several rhomboid insulin crystals. The A (α) cells, which constitute about 20 percent of the cells, secrete glucagon. They form a layer around the central core of B (β) cells and are identified ultrastructurally by their α granules, which are membrane-bound organelles with an electron-dense core and peripheral electron-lucent halo. The D (δ) and F cells are also found near the rim of the islets and are in close proximity to both A (α) and B (β) cells. The D (δ) cells secrete somatostatin and the F cells secrete pancreatic polypeptide. Somatostatin released locally affects the secretion of both the A and B cells, an example of paracrine regulation. The precise physiologic role of pancreatic polypeptide, which is secreted in response to protein-containing meals and has plasma levels similar to those of glucagon, is still uncertain. In addition to paracrine mechanisms, local communication between islet cells may also occur through "gap" junctions, direct contact points of the cell membranes of the different cell types.

Secretin is secreted by cells in the duodenal mucosa and regulates pancreatic exocrine secretion. It is responsible primarily for bicarbonate and fluid secretion.

Cardiovascular System: Blood Vessels

DIRECTIONS: Each question below contains five suggested responses. Select the **one best** response to each question.

86. Immediate compensatory reactions to hemorrhagic shock include

(A) decreased peripheral resistance
(B) constriction of the vessels of the brain and heart
(C) reduced levels of circulating catecholamines
(D) excessive loss of Na^+ in the urine
(E) none of the above

87. The largest portion of the arterial pressure generated during systole is dissipated at which of the following locations in the vascular tree?

(A) Aortic arch
(B) Aortic-arterial juncture
(C) Arterial-arteriolar juncture
(D) Arteriolar-capillary juncture
(E) Capillary-venular juncture

88. In which of the following organs will the rate of blood flow change the LEAST during exercise?

(A) Skin
(B) Brain
(C) Intestine
(D) Heart
(E) Kidney

89. Net movement of fluid from the intravascular space to the interstitial space occurs with all the following conditions EXCEPT

(A) constriction of postcapillary venules
(B) decreased plasma albumin concentration
(C) lymphatic obstruction
(D) constriction of precapillary arterioles
(E) activation of bradykinin

90. Venous pressure in the dural sinuses normally falls within which of the following ranges?

(A) Subatmospheric
(B) 0 to 5 mmHg
(C) 5 to 10 mmHg
(D) 10 to 20 mmHg
(E) Greater than 20 mmHg

91. Which of the following statements regarding the flow of blood through the vascular bed pictured below (the numbers are the radii) is true?

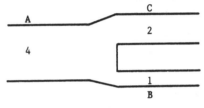

(A) The resistance of vessel C is two times the resistance of vessel A
(B) The resistance of vessel C is eight times the resistance of vessel A
(C) The flow through vessel C is twice the flow through vessel B
(D) The flow through vessel C is four times the flow through vessel B
(E) None of the above

92. From examination of the pressure-volume curve for the aorta illustrated below, which of the following conclusions can be drawn?

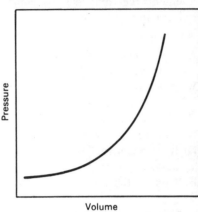

(A) The aorta is a high-capacitance vessel
(B) Aortic compliance increases as volume increases
(C) This curve reflects the behavior of the aorta only in an elderly person
(D) The collagen fibers in the aorta develop tension in proportion to their degree of elongation
(E) None of the above

93. Which one of the following characteristics is most similar in the systemic and pulmonary circulations?

(A) Stroke work
(B) Preload
(C) Afterload
(D) Peak systolic pressure
(E) Blood volume

94. If the concentration of a substance within capillary blood decreases linearly along the length of a capillary, which of the following statements regarding its movement from capillary blood to interstitial fluid is correct?

(A) It will increase if capillary flow increases
(B) It will increase if its plasma concentration increases
(C) It will decrease if plasma oncotic pressure decreases
(D) Its rate is inversely related to molecular size
(E) None of the above

95. Which of the following statements regarding closure of the ductus arteriosus is true?

(A) It reduces the flow of blood from the placenta to the vena cava
(B) It is stimulated by an increase in arterial P_{O_2}
(C) It interrupts a physiologic left-to-right shunt in the fetal circulation
(D) It is inhibited by prostacyclin
(E) None of the above

96. In general, the percentage of the cardiac output flowing to a particular organ is related to the metabolic activity of that organ in comparison with the other organs of the body. This relationship is true for all the following EXCEPT the

(A) brain
(B) heart
(C) skeletal musculature
(D) intestine
(E) kidney

97. The hemoglobin-oxygen saturation of blood entering the right ventricle is approximately

(A) 95 percent
(B) 85 percent
(C) 75 percent
(D) 55 percent
(E) 35 percent

98. All the following are likely to cause an increase in pulse pressure EXCEPT

(A) increasing stroke volume
(B) increasing diastolic pressure
(C) increasing aortic compliance
(D) increasing the rate of ventricular ejection
(E) increasing TPR (total peripheral resistance)

99. Occlusion of both carotid arteries between the heart and the carotid sinuses would be expected to produce

(A) increased blood pressure as measured in the femoral artery
(B) decreased heart rate
(C) increased activity in the afferent nerves from the carotid sinuses
(D) decreased activity of the vasomotor center
(E) decreased venous tone

100. Cerebral blood flow is influenced by all the following EXCEPT

(A) viscosity of the blood
(B) P_{O_2} of the arterial blood
(C) cerebrospinal fluid pressure
(D) pH of the interstitial fluid of the brain
(E) vasomotor reflexes

101. Which of the following changes in perfusion of an organ system is an example of autoregulation?

(A) The decrease in renal blood flow during hemorrhage
(B) The decrease in blood flow to the skin during exposure to a cold environment
(C) The increase in coronary perfusion during exercise
(D) The increase in cerebral blood flow during hypercapnia
(E) None of the above

102. The venous system can act as a reservoir for peripheral blood chiefly because of the

(A) low compliance of the venous wall
(B) absence of smooth muscle fibers in the venous wall
(C) superficial location of the veins
(D) large volume capacity of the venous system
(E) low oxygen saturation in the venous system

103. The greatest percentage of blood volume is found in the

(A) heart
(B) aorta
(C) distributing arteries and arterioles
(D) capillaries
(E) venules and veins

104. Lymph flow is increased by all the following EXCEPT

(A) elevated capillary pressure
(B) elevated plasma protein concentration
(C) elevated interstitial fluid protein concentration
(D) bradykinin
(E) exercise

105. Which of the following statements regarding activation of plasminogen is true?

(A) It follows a sequence of reactions involving serine proteases
(B) It occurs in blood but not in urine
(C) It is increased by vasodilatation
(D) It is inhibited by fibrin degradation products
(E) None of the above

106. *Diapedesis* is a term related to

(A) clotting
(B) pavementing
(C) cardiac arrest
(D) migration of neutrophils
(E) sickle cell anemia

107. Citrate is a useful anticoagulant because of its ability to

(A) buffer basic groups of coagulation factors
(B) bind factor XII
(C) bind vitamin K
(D) chelate calcium
(E) be slowly metabolized

108. Bleeding time is determined by nicking the skin superficially with a scalpel blade and measuring the time required for hemostasis. It will be markedly abnormal (prolonged) in a person who

(A) lacks factor VIII
(B) cannot absorb vitamin K
(C) has liver disease
(D) takes large quantities of aspirin
(E) takes coumarin derivatives

109. Lymph capillaries differ from systemic blood capillaries in that they

(A) are less permeable
(B) are not lined by endothelium
(C) lack valves
(D) are absent in the central nervous system
(E) collapse when interstitial pressure increases

110. In which of the following conditions will pulse pressure be higher than normal?

(A) Tachycardia
(B) Aortic stenosis
(C) Atherosclerosis
(D) Cardiac failure
(E) Mitral stenosis

111. Correct statements about the increase in pulmonary blood flow during vigorous exercise include which of the following?

(A) The percentage of increase in flow is greater in the bases of the lungs than in the apices
(B) The increase in flow is caused by a greater-than-fivefold increase in pulmonary arterial pressure
(C) The increase in pulmonary blood flow is less than the increase in systemic blood flow
(D) The increase in pulmonary blood flow is accommodated by dilation of pulmonary arterioles and capillaries
(E) The increase in pulmonary blood flow is caused by sympathetic nerve stimulation of the pulmonary vasculature

112. True statements concerning the activity of the baroreceptors of the carotid sinus include which of the following?

(A) It is increased by rapidly moving from a sitting to a standing position
(B) It is decreased by compression of the common carotid artery
(C) It produces an increase in total peripheral resistance
(D) It produces an increase in heart rate
(E) It produces an increase in stroke volume

113. Pulmonary lymph flow exceeds that in other tissues because

(A) pulmonary capillary pressure is higher than systemic capillary pressure
(B) pulmonary endothelial cells contain a large number of fenestrations
(C) alveolar epithelial cells secrete a fluid that is added to the lymph formed from the blood plasma
(D) pulmonary interstitial fluids contain more plasma proteins than the interstitial fluid in other tissues
(E) pulmonary capillaries have a lower oncotic pressure than systemic capillaries

114. Cerebral blood flow may be increased by increasing

(A) ventilation
(B) central venous pressure
(C) pH
(D) arterial blood pressure
(E) carbon dioxide tension

115. Neural control of circulation predominates over local control in which of the following organs?

(A) Brain
(B) Heart
(C) Skeletal muscle
(D) Kidney
(E) Skin

116. At birth, changes that occur in the fetal circulation include

(A) increased systemic arterial pressure
(B) increased pulmonary vascular resistance
(C) increased pulmonary arterial pressure
(D) decreased left atrial pressure
(E) decreased pulmonary blood flow

117. During vigorous exercise, blood flow in skeletal muscles increases tremendously because of which of the following factors?

(A) Circulating epinephrine dilates skeletal muscle blood vessels
(B) Activity of parasympathetic nerve fibers to the heart increases
(C) Resistance of the veins and venules decreases
(D) Total peripheral resistance increases
(E) None of the above

118. Hemorrhage generates all the following compensatory reactions EXCEPT

(A) arterial vasoconstriction
(B) venous vasoconstriction
(C) increased secretion of catecholamines
(D) bradycardia
(E) hemodilution

119. Turbulence is more likely to occur in a blood vessel if

(A) the velocity of blood within the vessel increases
(B) the viscosity of blood within the vessel increases
(C) the diameter of the vessel decreases
(D) the density of the blood decreases
(E) the length of the vessel increases

120. Arteriolar constriction may result from an increase in the local concentration of

(A) nitric oxide
(B) angiotensin II
(C) atrial natriuretic peptide
(D) beta agonists
(E) hydrogen ion

121. Hemorrhagic shock results in an increase in

(A) carbon dioxide tension
(B) anaerobic metabolism
(C) ventricular contractility
(D) cardiac output
(E) urine volume

122. All the following substances involved in platelet activation are derived from the platelets EXCEPT

(A) thrombin
(B) thromboxane A_2
(C) adenosine diphosphate
(D) prostaglandin H_2 (PGH$_2$)
(E) calcium

123. Increasing cytoplasmic calcium concentration within platelets stimulates

(A) activation of phospholipase C
(B) activation of phospholipase A_2
(C) elevation of cyclic-AMP concentration
(D) formation of protein kinase C
(E) inhibition of prostaglandin synthesis

124. The increase in viscosity associated with a decrease in blood velocity depends on

(A) the formation of red blood cell aggregates
(B) the tendency for red blood cells to migrate to the center of blood vessels
(C) an increase in the number of red blood cells that are unable to pass through the capillaries
(D) an increase in the concentration of red blood cells within the capillaries
(E) a decrease in the saturation of hemoglobin within the red blood cells

DIRECTIONS: Each group of questions below consists of lettered headings followed by several numbered items. For each numbered item select the **one** lettered heading with which it is **most** closely associated. Each lettered heading may be used **once, more than once, or not at all.**

Questions 125–129

The tracing shown below represents a normal jugular venous pulse. For each of the following statements, select the lettered point that it best describes.

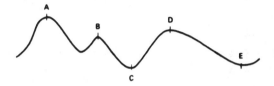

125. Reflects atrial systole

126. Becomes greatly amplified ("cannon wave") in patients with tricuspid stenosis

127. Increases in patients with tricuspid insufficiency

128. Results from bulging of tricuspid valve during ventricular systole

129. Is useful in distinguishing premature atrial contractions from premature ventricular contractions

Questions 130–132

The diagram below represents several sets of venous and cardiac function curves. The dashed curves labeled with a 1 are normal. Match each of the situations below with one of the letters corresponding to a point of intersection of a venous and cardiac function curve.

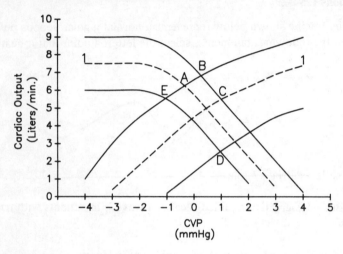

130. An increase in contractility

131. An increase in preload

132. A moderate hemorrhage

Cardiovascular System: Blood Vessels

Answers

86. The answer is E. *(Ganong, 15/e. pp 588–593.)* Loss of blood volume leads to generalized vasoconstriction, with the exception of the vessels of the brain and heart. Peripheral resistance increases, although in irreversible shock it may fall. Sympathetic discharge as well as increased adrenal medullary secretion contribute to the increase in circulating catecholamines. Elevated levels of circulating catecholamines probably contribute relatively little to the generalized vasoconstriction but may lead to stimulation of the reticular formation. Sodium retention is marked in hemorrhagic shock, a phenomenon that favors reexpansion of blood volume.

87. The answer is C. *(Ganong, 15/e. pp 541–543.)* The dissipation of a pulse wave in circulatory hemodynamics is most dependent on the diameter gradient between the proximal and distal vessels. Therefore, the greatest drop in pressure occurs at the level of branching where the difference in vessel diameters is the greatest. In the human, that is the arterial-arteriolar level.

88. The answer is B. *(West, 12/e. pp 155–156, 303–304.)* During exercise, metabolism and cardiac output increase. Blood flow to the skin increases to aid in the dissipation of heat while blood flow to the heart increases to provide adequate oxygen and nutrients and to remove wastes. During exercise, systemic resistance falls because of the extensive vasodilation in the exercising muscles. Blood flow to the intestine and kidney decreases in order to maintain adequate blood pressure. Autoregulatory mechanisms within the cerebral circulation keep blood flow in the brain from changing.

89. The answer is D. *(Ganong, 15/e. pp 545–546.)* The movement of fluid across the capillary wall is influenced by the transmural difference in hydrostatic and oncotic pressures, the permeability of the capillary wall, lymph flow, and the total volume of the extracellular fluid. Constriction of postcapillary venules would increase capillary hydrostatic pressure and force fluid out of the intravascular space, while constriction of precapillary arterioles would reduce capillary hydrostatic pressure. Reduced levels of plasma albumin such as occur in the nephrotic syndrome (increased loss of protein in the urine) or in hepatic cirrhosis (decreased protein synthesis) would reduce plasma oncotic pressure and favor net outward movement of fluid. Lymphatic obstruction leads to an increase in interstitial fluid volume by permitting interstitial fluid oncotic pressure to rise, though if edema becomes severe, interstitial fluid hydrostatic pressure also rises. Bradykinin increases net movement of fluid out of the capillary by increasing capillary permeability.

90. The answer is A. *(Ganong, 15/e. pp 548–549.)* Normal right atrial pressure is approximately 5 mmHg. Because of hydrostatic pressure, in the standing position venous pressure in the legs is greater than central venous pressure, whereas pressure in the head and neck is less. In the neck, normal veins collapse when a person is in an upright position; intracranially, the dural sinuses, having more rigid walls, are unable to collapse and sinus pressure may drop below 0 mmHg. During an intracranial operation upon a patient in a sitting position, the resultant negative pressure presents a danger that atmospheric air may be drawn into an exposed sinus and thus cause an air embolus.

91. The answer is E. *(Berne, 2/e. pp 474–480.)* Resistance of a blood vessel is proportional to $1/(radius)^4$. Since the radius of C is one-half the radius of A, it has 16 times the resistance of A. The flow through two vessels in parallel is proportional to 1/resistance. Since vessel C is twice the radius of B, it has $1/16$ the resistance and thus 16 times the flow.

92. The answer is E. *(Ganong, 15/e. pp 533–534. West, 12/e. pp 122–124.)* The pressure-volume curve illustrates the behavior of a large elastic vessel such as the aorta or main pulmonary artery. At lower volumes, pressure rises linearly as volume is increased because of the stretching of the abundant elastic fibers within the vessel wall. These fibers develop tension in proportion to the degree of stretching up to their limit. At higher volumes, where this limit is exceeded, pressure rises rapidly because the collagen fibers in the vessel wall are stiff and change very little in length with large changes in tension, thus causing a reduction in compliance as volume increases. This curve becomes even steeper (almost vertical) with age. In contrast to the aorta, large veins possess little elastic tissue and demonstrate a relatively flat pressure-volume curve. They are thus able to accommodate a large increase in volume with little change in pressure and are considered high-capacitance vessels.

93. The answer is B. *(West, 12/e. pp 112, 529–532.)* The right and left ventricles are in series with one another so that the entire cardiac output (except for a small anatomic shunt) passes through both circulations. Since the two ventricles beat at the same rate, their stroke volumes are the same. However, the resistance of the pulmonary vasculature is much smaller than that of the systemic circulation; thus the afterload and stroke work are greater on the left side than on the right side. Because the same cardiac output is ejected into a higher resistance, peak systolic pressure is higher on the left side than on the right side. Only about 10 percent of the blood volume is within the pulmonary circulation at any one time. About two-thirds of the blood volume is stored within the systemic veins and venules. Although the left and right preloads are not identical, they are very similar.

94. The answer is D. (*Ganong, 15/e. pp 545–546. West, 12/e. pp 128–131.*) Movement of substances across the capillary wall can occur by diffusion, filtration, or intracellular vesicular transport. Gases such as CO_2 and O_2, which are lipid-soluble, and small, water-soluble substances (e.g., glucose and urea) diffuse readily through the capillary wall, and their concentrations within capillary blood decrease rapidly with distance along the capillary because they equilibrate rapidly. Transcapillary movement of such substances will increase if their transcapillary concentration gradient increases or if capillary flow is increased. Transcapillary movement of larger molecules is dependent on filtration through the capillary pores and the rate of transcapillary movement is inversely related to their molecular size. Such substances do not reach equilibrium across the capillary, and their concentration decreases linearly along the length of the capillary.

95. The answer is B. (*Ganong, 15/e. pp 580–582. West, 12/e. pp 903–904.*) The ductus arteriosus connects the aorta and pulmonary artery and functions as a physiologic right-to-left shunt during fetal life because the lungs are collapsed and pulmonary vascular resistance is higher than systemic resistance. At birth, the lungs expand and pulmonary vascular resistance and pulmonary artery pressure fall drastically, while systemic vascular resistance and pressure rise owing to removal of the low-resistance placental circulation. Blood flow through the ductus is then reversed. Within a few hours the elevated P_{O_2} in the aortic blood passing through the ductus causes it to constrict and finally to close completely within a few weeks. When the ductus arteriosus fails to close spontaneously, surgical ligation may be necessary. Since the patency of the ductus is maintained in part by prostacyclin, inhibitors of prostaglandin synthesis such as indomethacin have been used to induce ductus closure and avoid surgery.

96. The answer is E. (*Ganong, 15/e. pp 570–578, 654–655.*) The kidney receives approximately 20 percent of the cardiac output while consuming a much smaller portion of the body's oxygen consumption. The high renal blood flow is related to the kidney's role in regulating the composition of the extracellular fluid. The skin is another organ in which the relationship between percentage of blood flow and percentage of oxygen consumption does not hold. Blood flow to the skin is primarily related to its role in temperature regulation. Of course in all organs, if oxygen consumption increases, blood flow will increase.

97. The answer is C. *(Ganong, 15/e. pp 616–618.)* The hemoglobin-oxygen dissociation curve is sigmoidal. Normally, P_{O_2} and hemoglobin saturation lie at the top of the curve so that hemoglobin saturation varies over a narrow range. Under physiologic conditions, the P_{O_2} of arterial blood is 100 mmHg and hemoglobin is approximately 98 percent saturated with oxygen. Some venous blood bypasses the lungs and prevents saturation from reaching 100 percent. Blood entering the right ventricle represents venous blood where P_{O_2} is at its lowest (40 mmHg) and hemoglobin saturation reaches its minimum of 75 percent.

98. The answer is C. *(Berne, 2/e. pp 490–492.)* Pulse pressure, the increase in arterial pressure during systole, is determined by the amount of blood added to the arterial system with each beat (called the volume increment) and the arterial compliance. The volume increment equals the stroke volume (the amount of blood ejected by the heart) minus the runoff (the amount of blood flowing from the arteries to the capillaries during systole). Increasing TPR will slow runoff, thus increasing the volume increment. Increasing the rate of ventricular ejection will increase the volume increment by increasing the rate at which blood is added to the arterial system. Increasing diastolic pressure may cause a decrease in aortic compliance and thus may cause an increase in pulse pressure. In contrast, increasing aortic compliance will always cause a decrease in pulse pressure.

99. The answer is A. *(Ganong, 15/e. pp 555–557.)* The carotid sinuses contain baroreceptors that respond to distention by discharging at an increased rate when arterial pressure rises. Impulses from these receptors inhibit the vasomotor center in the brainstem and cause vasodilatation. They also excite the cardioinhibitory center and cause bradycardia. Occlusion of the carotid arteries between the heart and the carotid sinuses would decrease the pressure in the sinus and remove the inhibitory influences on the brainstem, which in turn would result in tachycardia and vasoconstriction with increased arterial pressure.

100. The answer is E. *(Ganong, 15/e. pp 570–572.)* Cerebral blood flow is held constant under varying conditions. It is influenced by intracranial pressure, arterial pressure, arterial P_{O_2}, arterial and extracellular fluid pH, and blood viscosity. Vasomotor reflexes, mediated via the autonomic nervous system, have little part in controlling cerebral blood flow despite the fact that cerebral vessels are innervated by both sympathetic and parasympathetic fibers.

101. The answer is E. *(Ganong, 15/e. pp 550–551.)* Autoregulation is the maintenance of a constant blood flow in the presence of a change in arterial pressure. Two mechanisms have been used to explain autoregulation, the myogenic and metabolic theories. The myogenic theory proposes that an increase (or decrease) in perfusion pressure causes a contraction (or relaxation) of the arteriolar smooth muscle, thus reducing (or increasing) blood flow towards normal. The metabolic theory proposes that blood flow is adjusted to keep the concentration of metabolic by-products at a constant level. The changes in blood flow in response to overall homeostasis (e.g., the regulation of temperature or blood pressure during a hemorrhage) or specific tissue needs (e.g., the dilation of coronary arteries when the energy requirements of the heart increase during exercise) are not classified as autoregulatory processes.

102. The answer is D. *(Ganong, 15/e. pp 535, 541.)* The vessels of the venous system contain a thinner smooth muscle coat than their arterial and arteriolar counterparts but are still capable of significant contraction. The venous system has a large volume capacity. Thus, the level of tone within the system is important in the adjustment of blood volume in response to exercise and the gravitational effects of postural change.

103. The answer is E. *(Berne, 2/e. pp 395–397.)* The total circulating blood volume is approximately 70 mL/kg; about two-thirds is found in the systemic veins and venules. A significant volume of blood (15 percent) is found in the pulmonary circulation. Smaller quantities are found in the heart (5 percent), the arterial system (11 percent), and the capillaries (5 percent). The large volume of blood found on the venous side of the circulation is used to adjust circulating blood volume. For example, during hemorrhage, contraction of the veins and venules of the skin increases the amount of blood available for perfusion of the heart and brain.

104. The answer is B. *(Ganong, 15/e. pp 546–548. West, 12/e. pp 134–136.)* Lymphatic flow is essential for maintenance of a low interstitial fluid protein concentration and for prevention of fluid accumulation in tissues. The rate of lymph flow is regulated by the net interstitial fluid pressure and the pumping activity of the lymphatic vessels. Interstitial fluid pressure is normally subatmospheric because the colloid osmotic pressure of plasma that draws fluid into blood capillaries exceeds the sum of the capillary perfusion pressure and interstitial fluid pressure. When this balance is altered, interstitial fluid pressure rises to a level above atmospheric pressure and lymph flow is increased drastically. Imbalances may be caused by (1) elevated capillary pressure (cardiac failure); (2) increased interstitial fluid protein concentration, such as would occur following an increase in capillary permeability induced by bradykinin; or (3) decreased plasma oncotic pressure. Compression of lymphatic channels during exercise also promotes lymph flow. Increased plasma protein concentration would increase plasma colloid osmotic pressure and cause retention of fluid within capillaries.

105. The answer is C. *(West, 12/e. pp 397–398.)* Activation of plasminogen to plasmin, a serine protease that functions as the major fibrinolytic enzyme, occurs in both blood and urine by the action of different proteases. Vascular plasminogen activator is released from endothelial cells in response to stress, exercise, or vasodilatation and catalyzes the hydrolysis of plasminogen to plasmin while both are bound to a fibrin surface. It is rapidly cleared from the blood by the liver and has a half-life of only 15 min. Urokinase, the urinary plasminogen activator, catalyzes the cleavage in solution, thereby promoting fibrinolysis within renal tubules and preventing tubular occlusion. Cleavage of plasminogen to plasmin involves cleavage of a single arginine-valine bond. Fibrin degradation products released following fibrinolysis by plasmin inhibit hemostasis by interfering with the binding of fibrinogen to platelets.

106. The answer is D. *(Berne, 2/e. pp 362–364.)* Diapedesis is the process by which neutrophils pass through the endothelial layer and basement membrane of capillaries into surrounding tissue. Penetration of the vessel wall is preceded by margination and attachment of neutrophils to the capillary wall. This margination and migration occurs in response to chemotactic factors elaborated by bacteria or the immune system.

107. The answer is D. *(Ganong, 15/e. pp 501–502.)* The citrate ion has three anionic carboxylate groups that avidly chelate calcium and reduce the concentration of free calcium in blood. Because free calcium (Ca^{2+}) is required for multiple steps in both coagulation pathways, citrate is a useful anticoagulant in vitro. The citrate ion is rapidly metabolized; thus blood anticoagulated with citrate can be infused into the body without untoward effects. Oxalate, another calcium-chelating anticoagulant, is toxic to cells.

108. The answer is D. *(West, 12/e. pp 385–389.)* Hemostasis following blood vessel injury depends on (1) vascular spasm, (2) formation of a platelet plug, and (3) clot formation. When injury to a vessel produces only a small defect, the platelet plug itself can cause hemostasis. This is the basis for the bleeding time that is employed clinically to distinguish hemostatic abnormalities caused by platelet abnormalities from those caused by coagulation defects. Aspirin diminishes platelet aggregation by inhibiting cyclooxygenase, an enzyme required for generation of thromboxanes, which promote platelet aggregation. All the other situations described in the question are associated with coagulation deficiency. Persons thus affected would have a normal bleeding time but would present clinically with delayed posttraumatic bleeding caused by their inability to form an effective clot to reinforce the platelet plug.

109. The answer is D. *(West, 12/e. pp 131–133.)* Nearly all tissues of the body have a lymphatic circulation, one exception being the central nervous system. The lymphatic channels (or capillaries), which ultimately drain into the venous circulation, are lined by endothelial cells. These cells are attached to surrounding tissues by anchoring filaments and have large gaps between them to permit the free movement of macromolecules and particulate matter such as bacteria. The endothelial gaps are covered by overlapping, loosely adherent cell processes that act as valves to prevent the backflow of fluid once it enters the lumen. Valves, as well, exist within the channels every few millimeters to promote unidirectional flow.

110. The answer is C. *(Berne, 2/e. pp 490–492.)* Pulse pressure is the change in aortic pressure that occurs during systole. Anything that increases stroke volume or decreases aortic compliance will increase pulse pressure. Atherosclerosis is a disease of the arterial wall that causes an increased stiffness (or decreased compliance). Hypertension indirectly results in a decreased aortic compliance because of the nonlinearity of the aortic compliance curve; the greater the pressure within the aorta, the lower the compliance. In aortic stenosis and cardiac failure, stroke volume is either less than or equal to normal values and so pulse pressure does not increase.

111. The answer is D. *(Ganong, 15/e. pp 611–614.)* The pulmonary circulation is a low-pressure system compared with the systemic circulation. Because of this low pressure and the hydrostatic pressure gradient from the top, or apex, of the lung to the bottom, or base, of the lung, the apex of the lung is not as well perfused as the base of the lung. During vigorous exercise there is a large (up to sixfold) increase in cardiac output. The increased flow through the systemic circulation is equal to the increase in flow through the pulmonary circulation. Total lung flow increases and flow at the base of the lung is still greater than flow at the apex. However, the flow at the apex, since it was originally low, may increase by up to 800 percent, whereas flow in the base of the lung only increases by up to about 300 percent. The pulmonary vessels are very compliant. The increased flow causes recruitment of previously closed capillaries and dilation of pulmonary arterioles and capillaries. Because of this, pulmonary artery pressure normally does not increase or increases by only a small amount, and it rarely increases more than twofold.

112. The answer is B. *(Ganong, 15/e. pp 555–558.)* The carotid sinus is a specialized neural structure located in the wall of the internal carotid artery. It contains baroreceptors that respond to increases in arterial pressure; the receptors send signals to inhibit the vasoconstrictor center in the medulla and to excite the vagal center, which results in peripheral vasodilation and bradycardia. The carotid sinus also responds to sudden decreases in arterial pressure by relieving its inhibition of the vasoconstrictor center. For example, a decrease in baroreceptor activity is caused by the compression of the common carotid artery below the bifurcation (decreasing pressure in the sinus). Removing the inhibition from the vasoconstrictor and cardioaccelerator centers causes an increase in heart rate, ventricular contractility, and total peripheral resistance.

113. The answer is D. *(West, 12/e. pp 134–137.)* The rate of lymph flow is increased by factors that favor the flow of fluid from the capillaries to the interstitial spaces. Such factors include an elevation of capillary pressure, a decrease in plasma oncotic pressure, an increase in interstitial plasma proteins, and an increase in capillary permeability. The major factor involved in the increased formation of lymph within the lungs is the large leak of plasma proteins from the capillary to the interstitial fluid. The loss of plasma proteins from the capillaries occurs by diffusion through the spaces between capillary endothelial cells and not through endothelial cell fenestrations. The pressure within the pulmonary capillaries is lower than in systemic capillaries and so acts to reduce lymph formation. However, the negative intrapleural pressure acts to increase the pressure gradient across the capillary wall and so promotes lymph formation.

114. The answer is E. *(Ganong, 15/e. pp 570–571.)* Cerebral blood flow is under local metabolic control. The increase in H^+, CO_2, and K^+ that accompanies neural activity causes an increase in cerebral blood flow. Hyperventilation causes a respiratory alkalosis, which, by decreasing brain H^+ concentration (increasing pH), decreases cerebral blood flow. Increasing central venous pressure decreases the perfusion pressure across the brain vasculature and thus decreases cerebral blood flow. The brain is protected from an increase in blood flow during hypertension by autoregulatory mechanisms.

115. The answer is E. *(Ganong, 15/e. pp 567–571, 574–578.)* Blood flow to the skin is regulated by neuronal centers responsible for thermoregulation. Extensive sympathetic innervation of the AV anastomoses—particularly in the hands, feet, ears, and face—control the amount of blood flow through the skin. Neuronal innervation of the blood vessels to the brain, heart, and skeletal musculature is of secondary importance. In these organs, local metabolites (CO_2 and H^+ in the brain and skeletal muscles; adenosine in the heart) adjust blood flow to meet current metabolic needs. The kidney is largely under autoregulatory control, but under some circumstances, such as exercise or hemorrhage, the sympathetic nerve fibers innervating the renal blood vessels can shunt blood away from the kidney.

116. The answer is A. *(Ganong, 15/e. pp 581–582.)* At birth, two major events cause changes in the fetal circulation. First, loss of the placenta results in increased peripheral resistance and increased systemic arterial pressure. Second, expansion of the lungs allows marked pulmonary vasodilatation, which, by diminishing vascular resistance and promoting pulmonary blood flow, results in elevation of left atrial pressure.

117. The answer is E. *(Ganong, 15/e. pp 585–588.)* Blood flow to skeletal muscle increases by a factor of 15 to 20 during exercise because the exercising skeletal muscles release metabolites that dilate the arterioles within the muscles. Circulating catecholamines (norepinephrine and epinephrine) act to constrict blood vessels, not dilate them. In addition cardiac output increases and blood is shunted away from nonexercising muscles and other organs, such as the kidney and gastrointestinal tract, that can survive for the duration of exercise with a reduced blood flow. The massive dilation of blood vessels in exercising muscles is greater than the catecholamine-induced constriction in other organs and, as a result, total peripheral resistance decreases. Parasympathetic stimulation to the heart decreases during exercise, which allows the heart rate to increase. The veins and venules are constricted by sympathetic nerve discharge and circulating catecholamines. The increased tone within these muscles increases central venous pressure, which results in an increased preload and increased stroke volume.

118. The answer is D. *(Ganong, 15/e. pp 589–590.)* Reduction in blood volume by hemorrhage decreases venous return. The arterial baroreceptors are stretched to a lesser degree and sympathetic outflow is increased. There is reflex tachycardia and generalized vasoconstriction, except in the blood vessels of the brain and heart. Venoconstriction helps to maintain the filling pressure of the heart.

119. The answer is A. *(West, 12/e. pp 143–144.)* The critical factors affecting the flow of incompressible fluids in pipes were described late in the nineteenth century by the English physicist Osborne Reynolds. He discovered that the point at which flow changes from laminar (smooth) to turbulent is a function of fluid density, viscosity, and velocity and of the diameter of the vessel, expressed in the relationship that became known as the Reynolds number (Re):

$$ Re = \frac{density \times diameter \times velocity}{viscosity} $$

This relationship is equally valid for blood moving in the vessels of living organisms and for water moving in pipes. Increasing the length of the vessel may indirectly decrease the likelihood of turbulence by increasing vascular resistance and thus decreasing blood velocity.

120. The answer is B. *(Ganong, 15/e. pp 550–552.)* Angiotensin II is a powerful vasoconstrictor that is formed when renin is released from the kidney in response to a fall in blood pressure or vascular volume. Renin converts angiotensinogen to angiotensin I. Angiotensin II is formed from angiotensin I by an angiotensin-converting enzyme localized within the vasculature of the lung. All the other listed substances cause vasodilation.

121. The answer is B. *(Ganong, 15/e. pp 588–592.)* Hemorrhagic shock results from a massive loss of blood volume. The reduction in oxygen delivery to the tissues results in an increase in anaerobic metabolism and an increase in lactic acidosis. The decrease in pH in turn depresses the myocardium (decreases contractility). Blood is shunted away from the kidney so urine formation decreases or may even cease. The reduction in oxygen tension and the fall in pH stimulate the peripheral chemoreceptors, which by stimulating respiration cause a fall in carbon dioxide tension.

122. The answer is A. *(West, 12/e. pp 387–390.)* When platelets are exposed to a site of injury they are stimulated by thrombin and collagen. This stimulation activates (1) phospholipase C, which generates inositol triphosphate

(IP$_3$), which in turn releases calcium from internal stores; and (2) phospholipase A$_2$, which generates arachidonic acid, which is then oxidized by cyclooxygenase to produce thromboxane A$_2$ and PGH$_2$. Both of these amplify platelet activation: thromboxane A$_2$ enhances the action of collagen and PGH$_2$ increases the activity of phospholipase C. Adenosine diphosphate (ADP) is released from dense core granules within platelets. It enhances platelet activation.

123. The answer is B. *(West, 12/e. pp 387–390.)* Activation of platelets at a site of injury is stimulated by thrombin and the exposed collagen on the blood vessel endothelium. The activation process involves a G-protein–mediated activation of phospholipase C, which hydrolyzes phosphatidylinositol-4,5-bisphosphate (PIP$_2$) to form diacylglycerol (DAG) and IP$_3$. The IP$_3$, in turn, releases Ca^{2+} from internal stores. The elevated cytoplasmic Ca^{2+} concentration then leads to the activation of phospholipase A$_2$, which causes the release of arachidonic acid from the platelet membrane. Protein kinase C is activated by DAG. Prostaglandins, particularly PGH$_2$, are formed from arachidonic acid by a reaction catalyzed by cyclooxygenase.

124. The answer is A. *(West, 12/e. pp 139–141.)* The viscosity of blood depends on the hematocrit, the concentration of plasma proteins, and to some extent on the ability of red blood cells to undergo the deformation required for them to pass through the capillaries. The increase in viscosity caused by a decrease in velocity is related to the behavior of red blood cells. When the velocity of blood decreases, viscosity increases, and red blood cells tend to aggregate in stacks called *rouleaux*. Although red blood cells tend to migrate toward the center of blood vessels, this has the effect of lowering viscosity at low velocities. The lower viscosity occurs because most red blood cells remain in the larger branches when the stem vessel branches. The smaller number of red blood cells in the smaller vessels counteracts the increase in viscosity that normally accompanies a decrease in velocity.

125–129. The answers are: 125–A, 126–A, 127–B, 128–B, 129–A. *(Ganong, 15/e. p 524.)* Before the advent of echocardiography and other noninvasive techniques for assessing cardiac function, careful inspection of the jugular venous pulse was employed clinically to obtain significant information. Such information, although indirect, can still be derived from inspection.

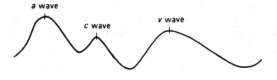

The jugular venous pressure wave reflects the changes in right atrial pressure that occur during the cardiac cycle. It normally consists of three positive pressure waves with intervening troughs. The first wave is the largest and is designated the *a* wave (answer A—see tracing accompanying questions). It reflects the rise in venous pressure owing to retrograde transmission of the force of atrial contraction during atrial systole when venous return is temporarily halted. The second peak (answer B) is termed the *c* wave and is produced by the bulging of the tricuspid valve into the atrium during the isometric ventricular contraction phase of ventricular systole. The tricuspid valve leaflets prevent backflow into the atrium and are assisted by contraction of the papillary muscles. The final wave of the venous pressure pulse (answer D) is termed the *v* wave. This increase in venous pressure occurs as the right atrium begins to fill during early diastole before the tricuspid valve opens.

In tricuspid insufficiency, the *c* wave becomes very large as the pressure of ventricular systole is transmitted through the incompetent valve to the superior vena cava. With tricuspid stenosis, where there is obstructed atrial emptying, venous pressure rises greatly during atrial contraction and produces a greatly amplified *a* wave. There would also be a slowing of the descent of the *v* wave. The jugular venous pressure is also influenced by alterations in cardiac rhythm. Premature atrial contractions can be distinguished from premature ventricular contractions because atrial contractions produce *a* waves and ventricular contractions do not. The *a-c* interval is nearly equal to the P-Q interval on the electrocardiogram and was used in the past as a measure of atrioventricular conduction.

130–132. The answers are: 130–A, 131–C, 132–E. *(Berne, 2/e. pp 525–534.)* The venous function curves represent the relationship between cardiac output (the independent variable) and right atrial pressure (the dependent variable). In general left ventricular preload is proportional to right atrial pressure (RAP), which in turn is proportional to central venous pressure (CVP). If cardiac output increases, RAP and preload decrease. Conversely, if cardiac output decreases, RAP and preload increase. The cardiac function curves represent the relationship between preload (the independent variable) and cardiac output (the dependent variable). This is the Starling relationship. The intersection of the two curves represents the value of the preload and cardiac output at any given time. If contractility increases, the cardiac function curve shifts up and to the left while the venous function curve remains the same. Thus, as represented by point A, there is an increase in cardiac output and a decrease in RAP. In order for preload to increase, circulating blood volume must increase. Thus, there is a parallel shift of the venous function curve to the right with no change in the cardiac function curve. This produces, as represented by point C, an increase in cardiac output and RAP. Hemorrhage is more complicated. Loss of blood produces a downward shift in the venous function curve. The response of the baroreceptor reflex to hemorrhage causes an increase in ventricular contractility, thus shifting the cardiac function curve up and to the left. Point E represents the cardiac output and preload that occur following a hemorrhage. Other responses to hemorrhage, such as a decrease in venous compliance and an increase in TPR, make the situation even more complicated. These effects are not represented on the diagram.

Cardiovascular System: Heart

DIRECTIONS: Each question below contains five suggested responses. Select the **one best** response to each question.

133. In a test subject, oxygen consumption was measured at 700 mL/min. Pulmonary artery oxygen content was 140 mL per liter of blood and brachial artery oxygen content was 210 mL per liter of blood. Cardiac output was which of the following?

(A) 4.2 L/min
(B) 7.0 L/min
(C) 10.0 L/min
(D) 12.6 L/min
(E) 30.0 L/min

134. Propagation of the action potential through the heart is slowest in the

(A) atrial muscle
(B) AV node
(C) His bundles
(D) Purkinje fibers
(E) ventricular muscle

135. Which of the following cardiac arrhythmias is LEAST likely to produce a change in the appearance of the QRS complex?

(A) First-degree heart block
(B) Second-degree heart block
(C) Third-degree heart block
(D) Atrial fibrillation
(E) Preventricular contraction

136. The greatest benefit derived from administering a positive inotropic drug to a patient in heart failure results from

(A) a reduction in heart rate
(B) a reduction in heart size
(C) an increase in contractile force
(D) an increase in wall thickness
(E) an increase in cardiac excitability

137. The electrocardiogram (ECG) is LEAST effective in detecting abnormalities in

(A) the position of the heart in the chest
(B) atrioventricular conduction
(C) cardiac rhythm
(D) cardiac contractility
(E) coronary blood flow

138. Impulses are conducted from the sinoatrial (SA) node of the heart to the atrioventricular (AV) node at an approximate rate of

(A) 0.1 millisecond (ms)
(B) 1.0 ms
(C) 0.1 second (s)
(D) 1.0 s
(E) 10.0 s

139. The repolarization phase of the cardiac cycle is represented by which portion of the ECG shown below?

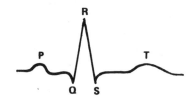

(A) P
(B) Q
(C) R
(D) S
(E) T

140. A decrease in stroke work is most likely to be caused by increasing

(A) contractility
(B) ejection fraction
(C) preload
(D) aortic compliance
(E) central venous pressure

141. The PR interval in an ECG is measured by finding the interval between the

(A) beginning of the P wave and the beginning of the R wave
(B) beginning of the P wave and the beginning of the QRS complex
(C) beginning of the P wave and the end of the QRS complex
(D) end of the P wave and the beginning of the QRS complex
(E) end of the P wave and the end of the QRS complex

142. Which of the following statements about second-degree heart block is correct?

(A) The PR interval is shortened
(B) The rate of ventricular contraction is increased
(C) Sinoatrial-atrioventricular (SA-AV) nodal conduction is slower
(D) AV nodal conduction is completely interrupted
(E) Not all atrial impulses reach the ventricles

143. At which point on the pressure volume curve illustrated below is the afterload on the heart the greatest?

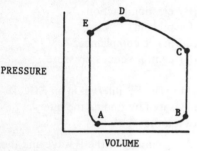

PRESSURE

VOLUME

(A) A
(B) B
(C) C
(D) D
(E) E

144. Closure of the aortic valve occurs at the onset of which phase of the cardiac cycle?

(A) Isovolumetric contraction
(B) Rapid ejection
(C) Protodiastole
(D) Isovolumetric relaxation
(E) Rapid filling

145. If the QRS complex is positive in lead II and negative in lead III, the mean electrical axis (MEA) is between

(A) −30 and +30
(B) +30 and +60
(C) +60 and +90
(D) +90 and +120
(E) +120 and +150

146. Patients who have received cardiac transplants are able to increase cardiac output during exercise for which of the following reasons?

(A) Heart rate is increased by sympathetic stimulation
(B) Ventricular end-diastolic pressure is decreased
(C) Increased venous return results in an increase in stroke volume
(D) Length of systole is shortened following transplantation
(E) None of the above

147. Mean left atrial pressure is normally greater than mean right atrial pressure for which of the following reasons?

(A) The diastolic pressure-volume curve for the right ventricle is steeper
(B) Left ventricular end-diastolic volume is greater
(C) The left atrium contains a smaller volume of blood
(D) The pulmonary veins are more compliant than the venae cavae
(E) None of the above

148. Coronary blood flow is increased by all the following EXCEPT

(A) beta-adrenergic blockade
(B) a decrease in arterial P_{O_2}
(C) an increase in arterial P_{CO_2}
(D) a decrease in systemic blood pressure
(E) vagal stimulation

149. A 6-month-old patient with a systolic murmur audible at the left sternal border could have any of the following abnormalities EXCEPT

(A) hyperthyroidism
(B) severe hemolytic anemia
(C) tricuspid stenosis
(D) congenital pulmonic stenosis
(E) patent foramen ovale

150. Persistence of a patent foramen ovale following birth does not cause significant physiologic abnormality because the

(A) left atrial pressure is higher than the right atrial pressure
(B) left ventricular output is greater than the right ventricular output
(C) left ventricular systolic pressure is greater than the right ventricular systolic pressure
(D) closure of the atrioventricular valves precedes ventricular ejection
(E) right atrial systole precedes left atrial systole

151. Splitting of the second heart sound (S_2) into two components is enhanced by

(A) delayed closure of the aortic valve
(B) delayed closure of the mitral valve
(C) early closure of the pulmonic valve
(D) prolongation of atrial systole
(E) none of the above

152. Which of the following statements about the third heart sound (S_3) is correct?

(A) It is usually diminished in congestive heart failure
(B) It is produced by turbulence during rapid ventricular filling in early diastole
(C) It is produced by turbulence following atrial contraction
(D) It is often associated with the "floppy" mitral valve syndrome
(E) It is produced by flow through the patent foramen ovale

153. In a resting, healthy man, the heart pumps how many liters of blood per minute?

(A) 0.9
(B) 2 to 3
(C) 5 to 6
(D) 8 to 10
(E) 15 to 20

154. Sustained elevation of cardiac output will occur with which of the following conditions?

(A) Hypertension
(B) Aortic regurgitation
(C) Anemia
(D) Third-degree heart block
(E) Cardiac tamponade

155. Based on the ECG below, the cardiac rhythm of the patient can be correctly described as

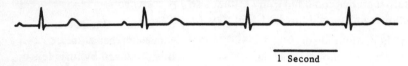

1 Second

(A) sinus arrhythmia
(B) first-degree heart block
(C) second-degree heart block
(D) atrial flutter
(E) tachycardia

156. The figure below indicates the relation between myocardial fiber length and left ventricular stroke work. The solid curve, which indicates the normal response of the heart to a work load, represents Starling's law of the heart. The dotted line indicates the response of a normal heart when something has been superimposed to alter the heart's response. On the basis of Starling's law, the dotted line could indicate

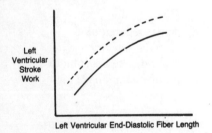

Left Ventricular End-Diastolic Fiber Length

(A) cardiac depression owing to hypoxia
(B) catecholamine response
(C) acetylcholine response
(D) congestive heart failure
(E) myocardial infarction

157. Which of the following will be greater during the plateau phase of the ventricular action potential than at rest?

(A) Sodium conductance
(B) Total membrane conductance
(C) Potassium conductance
(D) Calcium conductance
(E) Chloride conductance

158. Which one of the following statements concerning the mitral valve is correct?

(A) It requires contraction of the papillary muscle in order for it to close properly
(B) A systolic murmur is produced when it fails to close properly
(C) It closes at the end of isovolumic contraction
(D) It normally closes during the PR interval
(E) It prevents backflow of blood into the ventricle during diastole

159. All the following will help the heart to compensate for the reduction in contractility that occurs during heart failure EXCEPT an increase in

(A) retention of fluid by the kidney
(B) ventricular wall thickness
(C) sympathetic discharge
(D) end-diastolic volume
(E) total peripheral resistance

160. Increasing vagal stimulation of the heart will cause an increase in

(A) heart rate
(B) PR interval
(C) ventricular contractility
(D) ejection fraction
(E) cardiac output

161. During exercise there is an increase in a person's

(A) stroke volume
(B) diastolic pressure
(C) pulmonary arterial pressure
(D) pulmonary arterial resistance
(E) total peripheral resistance

162. If, under resting conditions, the heart rate is 70 beats per minute, the cardiac output is 5.6 L/min, and the end-diastolic volume is 160 mL, what is the ejection fraction?

(A) 0.40
(B) 0.45
(C) 0.50
(D) 0.55
(E) 0.60

163. Which of the following conditions will cause an increase in the size of the QRS complex recorded from lead II?

(A) A shift in the mean electrical axis from +60 degrees to 0 degrees
(B) Bradycardia
(C) Second-degree heart block
(D) Ventricular hypertrophy
(E) Mitral prolapse

164. Phase 4 depolarization of SA nodal cells is caused by

(A) an increase in the flow of sodium into the cell
(B) a decrease in the flow of potassium out of the cell
(C) an increase in the activity of the Na-Ca exchanger
(D) a decrease in the flow of chloride out of the cell
(E) a decrease in the activity of the Na-K pump

165. Cardiovascular changes that occur during inspiration include decreased

(A) right ventricular filling
(B) right ventricular output
(C) pressure gradient from extra-thoracic veins to the right atrium
(D) systemic arterial pressure
(E) left ventricular contractility

166. Blood pressure increases and heart rate decreases in response to

(A) exercise
(B) increased body temperature
(C) exposure to high altitude
(D) increased intracranial pressure
(E) hemorrhage

167. During exercise, cardiac output is augmented by

(A) sympathetic stimulation of resistance vessels
(B) dilation of venous vessels
(C) decreased end-diastolic volume
(D) decreased mean systemic arterial pressure
(E) increased ventricular contractility

168. When flow through the mitral valve is restricted by mitral stenosis,

(A) exercise can induce acute pulmonary edema
(B) left ventricular preload increases
(C) left atrial pressure diminishes
(D) right ventricular end-diastolic pressure decreases
(E) central venous pressure decreases

169. Stroke volume can be decreased by

(A) increasing ventricular contractility
(B) increasing heart rate
(C) increasing central venous pressure
(D) decreasing total peripheral resistance
(E) decreasing systemic blood pressure

170. An average man at rest has a stroke volume that is

(A) greater from the left ventricle than from the right ventricle
(B) equal to the cardiac output divided by the heart rate
(C) independent of body surface area
(D) approximately 150 mL
(E) independent of the preload

171. All the following increase as the heart compensates for aortic regurgitation EXCEPT

(A) left ventricular end-diastolic volume
(B) left ventricular stroke volume
(C) ventricular mass
(D) pulse pressure
(E) net cardiac output

172. An ectopic extrasystole caused by a ventricular focus is characterized by

(A) interruption of the regular SA node discharge
(B) retrograde conduction of the action potential to the atrium
(C) a skipped ventricular contraction
(D) a skipped atrial contraction
(E) a larger-than-normal force of contraction

DIRECTIONS: Each group of questions below consists of lettered headings followed by a set of numbered items. For each numbered item select the **one** lettered heading with which it is **most** closely associated. Each lettered heading may be used **once, more than once, or not at all.**

Questions 173–177

The phases of the action potential of ventricular muscle are represented by the lettered points on the diagram. Match each of the events listed below with the phase with which it is most closely associated.

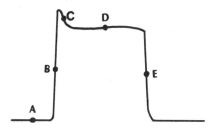

173. Activation of sodium channels

174. An increase in calcium conductance

175. Inactivation of sodium channels

176. Activation of potassium channels

177. A decrease in potassium conductance

Questions 178–182

Match the events in the cardiac cycle with the time points in the pressure tracings below. If no time point corresponds to the event listed, select E.

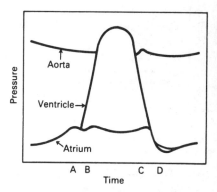

178. Onset of isovolumetric ventricular contraction

179. Closure of aortic valve

180. Opening of mitral valve

181. Completion of atrial systole

182. Onset of ventricular repolarization

Questions 183–186

For each condition listed, select the lettered point on the Frank-Starling curves shown below with which it is most likely to be associated. (Assume point C is the resting state.)

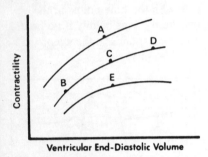

Ventricular End-Diastolic Volume

183. Acute volume overload

184. Metabolic acidosis

185. Pericardial effusion

186. Muscular exercise

Questions 187–190

For each circumstance listed below, select the effect on heart rate and blood pressure that it is most likely to have.

(A) Heart rate increased, blood pressure increased

(B) Heart rate increased, blood pressure decreased

(C) Heart rate decreased, blood pressure decreased

(D) Heart rate decreased, blood pressure increased

(E) No change in heart rate and blood pressure

187. Increased intracranial pressure

188. Syncope

189. Hypoxia

190. Exercise

Cardiovascular System: Heart

Answers

133. The answer is C. *(Ganong, 15/e. pp 526–527.)* Cardiac output can be measured by using the Fick principle, which asserts that the rate of uptake of a substance by the body (e.g., O_2 consumption in milliliters per minute) is equal to the difference between its concentrations (milliliters per liter of blood) in arterial and venous blood multiplied by the rate of blood flow (cardiac output). This principle is restricted to situations in which arterial blood is the only source of the substance measured. If oxygen consumption by the body at steady state is measured over a period of time and the difference in arterial O_2 and venous O_2 measured by sampling arterial blood and *pulmonary* arterial blood (which is fully mixed venous blood), cardiac output is obtained from the expression

$$\text{cardiac output} = \frac{O_2 \text{ consumption (mL/min)}}{[(A_{O_2}) - (V_{O_2})] \text{ (mL/L)}}$$

Substituting the values for the test subject presented in the question,

$$\text{cardiac output} = \frac{700}{210 - 140} = 10 \text{ L/min}$$

134. The answer is B. *(Ganong, 15/e. p 506.)* The propagation of the action potential through the heart is fastest in the His-Purkinje network. The high speed of conduction ensures that the entire ventricle will be depolarized at the same time. The slowest speed of conduction is within the AV node. The delay in propagation between the atria and ventricles provides time for the blood ejected from the atria during atrial systole to enter the ventricles before the ventricles contract.

135. The answer is A. *(Ganong, 15/e. pp 510–516.)* The QRS complex represents the depolarization of the ventricles. Under normal circumstances, the ventricles are depolarized by the propagation of the action potential along the

His-Purkinje system. Anything that interferes with the normal propagation pathway will cause the QRS complex to appear abnormal. In principle, the QRS complex can appear normal under all the listed situations if the common bundle branch is the first part of the ventricle to depolarize. However, this is unlikely to happen when the action potential does not pass along its normal path from the atria to the ventricles. The pathway is least likely to be interrupted in a first-degree heart block.

136. The answer is B. (*West, 12/e. pp 258–259, 307–312.*) The most obvious deleterious effect of a failing heart is the inability to pump enough blood to satisfy the energy requirements of all the tissues. Among the compensatory mechanisms that develop in response to heart failure is an increase in retention of fluid by the kidney. Increased retention of fluid causes the end-diastolic volume of the heart to increase, which, by the Starling mechanism, increases the strength of the heart beat. However, two deleterious effects result from an increase in end-diastolic volume. A larger-than-normal end-diastolic volume causes an increase in end-diastolic pressure, which can lead to pulmonary edema. In addition, the large end-diastolic volume increases the wall stress that must be developed by the heart with each beat, and this increases the myocardial requirement of oxygen. The increase in contractility that results from the administration of a positive inotropic drug such as ouabain will allow the heart to produce the same force at a lower volume and thus eliminate the need for an increase in volume of fluid.

137. The answer is D. (*Berne, 2/e. pp 409–429.*) The ECG records the conduction of the action potential through the heart. Changes in the rate, rhythm, or conduction pathway are recorded. Changes in the position of the heart in the chest will change the size and shape of the ECG recorded by the various leads. Local areas of ischemia caused by changes in coronary blood flow will cause changes in the action potentials that will be reflected in the shape of the ECG recording. The ECG is unable to detect any changes in the ability of the heart to develop force.

138. The answer is C. (*Ganong, 15/e. p 506.*) One-tenth of a second is the order of magnitude to remember when thinking of the rate of cardiac depolarization. Atrial depolarization is completed in 0.08 to 0.1 s, followed by a 0.1-s atrioventricular (AV) nodal delay. Ventricular depolarization is then completed in 0.08 to 0.1 s.

139. The answer is E. (*West, 12/e. pp 177, 181–182, 186–187.*) In the electrocardiogram (ECG) that appears with the question, the section representing the repolarization phase of the cardiac cycle is labeled T, corresponding to the T wave of the ECG. It is a positive deflection and represents the return of relative negativity to the cardiac muscle. The P wave represents atrial depolarization, and points Q, R, and S collectively represent a complex corresponding to ventricular depolarization. Atrial repolarization deflections normally are hidden in the QRS complex.

140. The answer is D. *(West, 12/e. pp 292–296.)* Stroke work is the product of stroke volume and mean systolic pressure. Increasing contractility, ejection fraction, and preload will all cause an increase in stroke volume and pressure. Thus stroke work will increase. Increasing central venous pressure results in an increase in preload so it, too, will cause an increase in stroke work. Increasing aortic compliance will cause a decrease in the rise in pressure during ejection, and so stroke work will decrease.

141. The answer is B. *(Ganong, 15/e. pp 506–508.)* The PR interval in an ECG is measured from the beginning of the P wave, which reflects atrial depolarization, to the beginning of the QRS complex, which reflects initiation of ventricular depolarization. This interval normally ranges from 0.12 to 0.2 s and reflects the time required for atrial depolarization and conduction through the atrioventricular node. The PR interval is prolonged by vagal stimulation and hypokalemia and shortened by sympathetic stimulation.

142. The answer is E. *(West, 12/e. pp 195–196.)* Blockade of conduction through the atrioventricular node or infranodal ventricular conduction system affects the transmission of atrial impulses to the ventricles. In first-degree heart block, the PR interval is prolonged, but all atrial impulses are transmitted to the ventricles. In second-degree heart block, the PR interval is prolonged, but some of the atrial impulses are not passed through the atrioventricular node, so that the ventricles beat at a slower rate than the atria. Third-degree or complete heart block occurs when atrioventricular or infranodal conduction is completely interrupted and the ventricles beat at a much slower rate driven by their own intrinsic rhythm.

143. The answer is C. *(West, 12/e. pp 223–228.)* Although afterload is sometimes considered equal to the ventricular pressure, wall stress is a truer measure of afterload. Wall stress is proportional to (pressure × radius) / wall thickness. It is greatest at C, where the radius is greater than it is at D. The lower pressure at C does not make up for the greater radius.

144. The answer is D. *(Ganong, 15/e. pp 521–526.)* Closure of the semilunar valves (aortic and pulmonic valves) marks the beginning of the isovolumetric relaxation phase of the cardiac cycle. During this brief period (approximately 0.06 s), the ventricles are closed and myocardial relaxation, which began during protodiastole, continues. Intraventricular pressure falls rapidly, although ventricular volume changes little. When intraventricular pressure falls below atrial pressure, the mitral and tricuspid valves open and rapid filling of the ventricles begins.

145. The answer is A. *(Berne, 2/e. pp 422–424.)* If the QRS complex is positive in lead II, the MEA must be between −30 and +120. If the QRS complex is negative in lead III, the MEA must be between −150 and +30. For both conditions to exist, the MEA must be between −30 and +30.

146. The answer is C. *(Ganong, 15/e. pp 530–531.)* During exercise, normal persons experience an increased sympathetic discharge that increases both myocardial contractility and heart rate so that cardiac output increases with little increase in stroke volume. In cardiac transplant patients whose hearts have been denervated, direct sympathetic stimulation does not occur. Cardiac output increases by the operation of the Frank-Starling mechanism. Thus, the increased venous return that occurs during exercise results in an increase in ventricular end-diastolic pressure. In turn, myocardial contractility and stroke volume increase.

147. The answer is C. *(Berne, 2/e. pp 461–462.)* Left atrial pressure is higher than right atrial pressure during all phases of the cardiac cycle. Two factors contribute to this difference. The wall of the right ventricle is thinner than that of the left ventricle and is less stiff (more compliant); consequently, when atrial contraction forces equal volumes of blood into the ventricles, left ventricular end-diastolic pressure (and thus left atrial end-diastolic pressure) is greater because the left ventricle has a steeper diastolic pressure-volume curve, i.e., a greater change in pressure for the same change in volume. In addition, the pulmonary veins and left atrium contain a smaller volume and are less compliant than the venae cavae and right atrium. Thus, when equal volumes of blood enter the atria during ventricular systole, left atrial pressure rises to a higher level than right atrial pressure.

148. The answer is A. *(Ganong, 15/e. pp 574–575. West, 12/e. pp 267–272.)* Because the heart functions at maximal levels of oxygen extraction even at rest, coronary blood flow must increase when myocardial oxygen demand is increased. Coronary blood flow is regulated by both chemical and neural factors. Decreased arterial P_{O_2} and increased P_{CO_2} both increase coronary blood flow even in denervated hearts. Both vagal and beta-adrenergic stimulation result in coronary vasodilatation. When systemic blood pressure falls, reflex noradrenergic stimulation causes an increase in coronary blood flow and renal splanchnic and cutaneous vasoconstriction. When beta-adrenergic receptors are blocked, noradrenergic stimulation mediated by alpha-adrenergic receptors results in coronary vasoconstriction.

149. The answer is E. *(Ganong, 15/e. pp 525–526.)* Murmurs are abnormal sounds produced by turbulent blood flow caused by an obstruction or by rapid flow through a narrow orifice. The location of cardiac murmurs caused by valvular disease can often be determined by their timing in the cardiac cycle. For example, aortic or pulmonic stenosis produces a systolic murmur, whereas tricuspid or mitral stenosis produces a diastolic murmur because those are the phases of the cycle when flow occurs through those orifices. Patients with hyperthyroidism or anemia will also have systolic murmurs caused by increased flow or decreased viscosity, respectively. With a patent foramen ovale (atrial septal defect), even if the defect is large, no murmur is audible because of the low pressure differential (1 to 3 mmHg) between left and right atria.

150. The answer is A. *(West, 12/e. pp 903–906.)* In the fetus, the foramen ovale permits most of the oxygenated blood returning to the right atrium to bypass the unoxygenated pulmonary circulation and pass directly into the left atrium, thence into the left ventricle from which the blood is ejected into the systemic circulation via the aorta. The foramen ovale is normally covered by a valvelike leaflet that prevents backflow. At birth, owing to loss of the placental blood flow, there is an increase in systemic vascular resistance, which increases the pressure in the aorta and left atrium, and as the lungs expand there is a decrease in pulmonary vascular resistance, which decreases the pressure in the pulmonary artery and right atrium. Anatomic closure of the foramen ovale prevents left-to-right shunting, although even without closure the pressure gradient between atria is sufficient to keep the valve functionally closed.

151. The answer is E. *(West, 12/e. pp 239–241.)* The second heart sound (S_2) is produced by vibrations in the arterial blood column and arterial walls as the aortic and pulmonic valves undergo tension during closure. Heard over the left sternal border, this sound normally can be resolved into two components representing closure of the aortic and pulmonic valves. Resolution is greatest during inspiration, when venous return increases on the right and prolongs right ventricular ejection. Any event that delays closure of the pulmonic valve thus enhances the splitting; delayed closure of the aortic valve or early closure of the pulmonic valve diminishes the splitting. Closure of the mitral valve and atrial systole influence the first heart sound (S_1).

152. The answer is B. *(West, 12/e. pp 239–241.)* The third heart sound (S_3), also termed the *ventricular diastolic gallop*, is produced by turbulence occurring during the initial phase of rapid ventricular filling in diastole. It may be heard normally in younger persons but is usually louder in patients with congestive heart failure where ventricular compliance is reduced. Turbulence during ventricular filling following atrial contraction at the end of diastole gives rise to the atrial diastolic gallop or fourth heart sound (S_4), also associated with decreased ventricular compliance. Flow through a patent foramen ovale is silent because there is little turbulence in the low-pressure atria.

153. The answer is C. *(Ganong, 15/e. pp 527–528.)* Cardiac output is determined by the product of the stroke volume and heart rate. At rest, stroke volume is about 80 mL and heart rate is 70 beats per minute. Thus, cardiac output would be 5 to 6 L/min in the average healthy man; in the average healthy woman, it is 10 to 20 percent less. Cardiac output can increase several-fold during exercise and would be decreased in the presence of depressed myocardial function and reduced stroke volume, or in the presence of arrhythmias that alter heart rate.

154. The answer is C. *(West, 12/e. pp 315–319.)* The magnitude of the cardiac output is regulated to maintain an adequate blood pressure and to deliver an adequate supply of oxygen to the tissues. In anemia, a greater cardiac output is required to supply oxygen to the tissues because the oxygen-carrying capacity of the blood is reduced. In aortic regurgitation, the stroke volume will be increased. However, a portion of the blood ejected by the heart will return to the heart during diastole. Thus the output delivered to the tissues does not increase despite the fact that the blood ejected by the heart has increased. In hypertension, third-degree heart block, and cardiac tamponade (decreased filling of the heart due to accumulation of fluid within the pericardium), cardiac output will be normal or, if compensation is not possible, cardiac output will be reduced.

155. The answer is B. *(Berne, 2/e. pp 424–429. West, 12/e. pp 189–196.)* The normal PR interval is between 0.12 and 0.2 s. In this ECG, the PR interval is 0.25 s and thus the patient has a first-degree heart block. The heart rate is 40 beats per minute, which is a bradycardia; a tachycardia is a heart rate above 100 beats per minute. There is no sign of any rhythm disturbance such as sinus arrhythmia or atrial flutter.

156. The answer is B. *(Ganong, 15/e. pp 528–531.)* The Starling principle states that increasing venous return (which increases fiber length) increases cardiac output and stroke work. The dotted line appearing in the graph that accompanies the question indicates a situation in which more work is done for the *same* length of fiber stretch than occurs normally with a work load. Stimulation of the heart by a catecholamine, like epinephrine, would represent such a situation. Heart disease and acetylcholine, on the other hand, by diminishing the heart's pumping capacity, would produce a curve *below* that of the normal Frank-Starling curve.

157. The answer is D. *(Berne, 2/e. pp 398–406.)* During the plateau phase of the cardiac action potential, potassium conductance decreases below its resting value while calcium conductance is greater than it is at rest. However, the decrease in potassium conductance is greater than the increase in calcium conductance, so total membrane conductance decreases. The sodium channels inactivate during the plateau phase, returning sodium conductance to its resting value.

158. The answer is B. *(West, 12/e. pp 115–117, 239–242.)* The mitral valve is situated between the left ventricle and left atrium and acts to prevent the flow of blood from the ventricle to the atrium during isovolumic contraction. If the valve fails to close properly, blood will flow into the atrium during ventricular contraction and produce a systolic murmur. The valve normally closes at the beginning of isovolumic contraction, which occurs after the QRS complex has begun rather than within the PR interval. Contraction of the papillary muscles pulls on the chordae tendineae, which prevents the mitral valve from being pushed too far into the atrium during ventricular contraction. However, the papillary muscles do not contribute to the closing of the valve.

159. The answer is E. *(West, 12/e. pp 307–312.)* When the heart fails, either because of cardiac disease or inadequate oxygen delivery, its output is reduced. The decrease in cardiac output is sensed by the regulatory processes controlling renal volume excretion, which respond by retaining fluid. The increase in fluid helps restore cardiac output to normal by enhancing venous return and increasing end-diastolic volume. The reduction in cardiac output also causes a decrease in blood pressure. The decrease in blood pressure stimulates the baroreceptor reflex, which increases sympathetic stimulation. The increase in sympathetic stimulation in turn increases cardiac output directly by increasing the force of each heart beat and indirectly by increasing venous return. However, sympathetic stimulation also increases total peripheral resistance (TPR), which makes it more difficult for the heart to eject blood. Ventricular wall thickness (ventricular hypertrophy) increases as a long-term compensation in cardiac failure. The thicker wall increases the force-generating capability of the ventricle.

160. The answer is B. *(Berne, 2/e. pp 451–452.)* The vagal fibers innervating the heart stimulate intracardiac postganglionic fibers, which release acetylcholine (ACh). The postganglionic fibers innervate the SA and AV nodal fibers. ACh causes a decrease in the rate of phase 4 depolarization, thus slowing the heart, and a decrease in conduction velocity through the AV node, thus increasing the PR interval. ACh also causes a slight decrease in contractility. Decreasing the heart rate increases the amount of time available for ventricular filling and thus increases end-diastolic volume. However, the end-systolic volume will be somewhat elevated because of the slight decrease in contractility and increase in afterload. Thus, the ejection fraction will remain the same or decrease slightly.

161. The answer is A. *(West, 12/e. pp 304–306.)* During exercise, increased oxygen consumption and increased venous return to the heart result in an increase in cardiac output and an increase in blood flow to both skeletal muscle and the coronary circulation, where oxygen utilization is greatest. The increase in cardiac output is due to an increase in both heart rate and stroke volume. Systemic arterial pressure also increases in response to the increase in cardiac output. However, the fall in total peripheral resistance, which is caused by dilation of the blood vessels within the exercising muscles, results in a decrease in diastolic pressure. The pulmonary vessels undergo passive dilation as more blood flows into the pulmonary circulation. As a result, pulmonary vascular resistance decreases and pulmonary blood volume increases as cardiac output increases. Pulmonary artery pressure may increase if the increase in cardiac output is unusually large.

162. The answer is C. *(Guyton, 8/e. p 103.)* The ejection fraction is defined as the stroke volume divided by the end-diastolic volume. If the cardiac output is 5.6 L/min and the heart rate is 70 beats per minute, then the stroke volume is 5600 / 70 = 80 mL. The ejection fraction is thus 80 / 160 = 0.50.

163. The answer is D. *(Berne, 2/e. pp 422–426.)* The magnitude of the QRS complex depends on the mass of tissue depolarized, the closeness of the ventricle to the recording electrode, and the relationship between the direction of ventricular depolarization and the orientation of the recording leads. Ventricular hypertrophy increases the magnitude of the QRS complex in all leads.

When the mean electrical axis is horizontal, the size of the QRS complex in lead I increases while that in leads II and III diminishes. Although slowing of the heart rate may increase the force of contraction, it has no effect on the size of the QRS complex. In second-degree heart block, the ventricular beats that do occur have QRS complexes of normal shape.

164. The answer is A. *(Berne, 2/e. pp 410–413.)* Phase 4 depolarization is caused by the activation of two currents: a sodium current and a calcium current. The sodium current is activated when the cell repolarizes. The greater the repolarization, the greater the sodium current. Because of the unusual way in which this current is activated, it is called the *funny current* (i_f). The calcium current is activated near the end of phase 4 depolarization. The calcium current flows through a slowly activated channel and is called the i_{si}. Potassium conductance decreases during phase 4 depolarization and thus the flow of potassium out of the cell is diminished. However, this change in potassium current is not responsible for phase 4 depolarization. Chloride conductance does not change during phase 4. Changes in chloride conductance are not involved in the cardiac action potential. The Na-Ca exchanger maintains low intracellular calcium at rest and may reverse its direction and pump calcium into the cell during phase 2 of the cardiac action potential. However, neither the Na-Ca exchanger nor the Na-K pump is involved in phase 4 depolarization.

165. The answer is D. *(West, 12/e. pp 232–233.)* Because intrathoracic pressure is reduced during inspiration, the pressure gradient from the extrathoracic to intrathoracic veins increases and right ventricular filling and right ventricular output increase. However, pulmonary venous return is decreased by the reduction in intrathoracic pressure. This produces a decrease in *left* ventricular stroke volume, which results in a decrease in systemic arterial pressure.

166. The answer is D. *(Ganong, 15/e. pp 102, 285, 288–289.)* Exercise increases blood pressure and heart rate. Although tissue hypoxia causes arteriolar dilatation, acute hypoxia associated with sudden exposure to high altitudes generates hypertension, as well as excitement, disorientation, and headache. Fever produces tachycardia; blood pressure changes associated with increased body temperature depend on the cause of the temperature. With exercise and increased heat production (and increased blood pressure), vessels dilate in an attempt to dissipate heat. Fever with septic shock will, of course, be associated with a blood pressure decrease owing to vasodilatation by endotoxin. Hemorrhage will cause a reflex sympathetic discharge that results in tachycardia and increased total peripheral resistance. If compensation is adequate, blood pressure may not fall. If intracranial pressure is rapidly elevated, cerebral blood flow is reduced. The resulting hypoxia stimulates the vasomotor center and produces an increase of systemic blood pressure and restoration of cerebral blood flow (Cushing's law). There is reflex bradycardia and decreased respiratory rate.

167. The answer is E. *(Ganong, 15/e. pp 530–531, 585–587.)* During exercise, sympathetic stimulation of the heart and circulating epinephrine cause an increase in ventricular contractility and heart rate leading to an increase in cardiac output. Sympathetic stimulation also causes constriction of the venous vessels, which tends to increase end-diastolic volume. Despite sympathetic stimulation of the resistance vessels, local metabolites cause three small arterioles to dilate, which produces a decrease in total peripheral resistance (TPR). However, the fall in TPR does not normally produce a drop in mean systemic blood pressure because the increase in cardiac output is sufficient to counteract the fall in resistance.

168. The answer is A. *(West, 12/e. pp 242, 307.)* In patients with mitral stenosis, the flow of blood from the left atrium to left ventricle during diastole is diminished. The left atrium progressively dilates and left atrial pressure rises. The increase in pressure is transmitted through the pulmonary circulation and eventually leads to an increase in right ventricular pressure. When cardiac output increases during exercise, restriction to flow through the mitral valve causes a sudden increase in pulmonary blood volume, and pulmonary venous and capillary pressures rise, which leads to transudation of fluid into alveoli and pulmonary edema.

169. The answer is B. *(West, 12/e. pp 227–232.)* Stroke volume is determined by preload, afterload, and contractility. Increasing preload by increasing central venous pressure will increase stroke volume. Similarly, decreasing afterload by decreasing total peripheral resistance or systemic blood pressure will cause an increase in stroke volume. Increasing contractility will also increase stroke volume. Cardiac output equals stroke volume times heart rate. If the heart rate increases and cardiac output does not change, stroke volume will decrease.

170. The answer is B. *(Ganong, 15/e. pp 527–531.)* The normal cardiac output of an average man is 5.5 L/min. Thus, his stroke volume is

$$\frac{5.5 \text{ L/min}}{70 \text{ beats/min}} = 78.5 \text{ mL}$$

Cardiac output varies with body surface area; the output per minute per square meter of body surface, which is known as the *cardiac index,* averages about 3.2 L. The stroke volume of the right ventricle must equal the stroke volume of the left, in the absence of pathologic shunting. If preload changes, the stroke volume will change proportionally.

171. The answer is E. *(West, 12/e. p 315.)* In aortic regurgitation, much of the blood ejected during systole reenters the left ventricle during diastole. The ventricle dilates and the end-diastolic volume is increased. The left ventricular stroke volume has to be increased to handle the blood normally entering from the atrium in addition to the blood that returns from the aorta. The net cardiac output is thus normal or decreased. The pulse pressure is widened because of the elevated systolic pressure (brought about by the increased stroke volume) and reduced diastolic pressure (as a consequence of backflow of blood through the incompetent aortic valve). The increased volume load on the heart causes ventricular hypertrophy.

172. The answer is C. *(Ganong, 15/e. pp 514–515.)* A premature heartbeat, or ectopic extrasystole, places the myocardium in a refractory period at the time of arrival of the next normal stimulus from the SA node. Therefore, no ventricular contraction can occur. The impulse from the ectopic focus is incapable of exciting the bundle of His and thus no retrograde conduction to the atrium takes place. Inasmuch as the ectopic event does not extend to the atrium, the atrium continues to contract regularly under the influence of the SA node. The ventricular contraction is smaller because the heart has not filled to its normal end-diastolic volume when the extrasystole occurs. In addition, the extrasystole does not propagate normally through the ventricle so the force of contraction is reduced.

173–177. The answers are: 173-B, 174-D, 175-C, 176-E, 177-D. *(Berne, 2/e. pp 401–406.)* The action potential of the ventricular muscle is initiated when the membrane potential is depolarized to threshold. At threshold, sodium channels are activated, which increases the flow of sodium into the cell. The flow of sodium into the cell causes further depolarization, which in turn causes more sodium channels to become activated, which again results in more sodium flow into the cell. This regenerative process causes the rapid upstroke of the action potential (phase 0, point B). Membrane depolarization causes inactivation of the sodium channels and is responsible for the small phase 1 repolarization (point C). Inactivation of sodium channels, however, does not cause the membrane to return to its resting potential. Instead the membrane remains depolarized, producing the plateau phase (phase 2) of the action potential. Phase 2 (point D) is associated with an increase in calcium conductance and a decrease in potassium conductance. The increase in calcium conductance is caused by the opening of calcium channels. The amount of calcium entering the cell during the plateau phase influences the strength of the heart beat. Norepinephrine increases contractility by increasing the flow of calcium into the cell. Various calcium blocking agents, such as nifedipine and verapamil, decrease contractility by diminishing the amount of calcium entering the ventricular cells. The decrease in potassium conductance is not as well understood. It is called *anomalous rectification* to distinguish it from the delayed rectification (or increase in potassium conductance) that causes the repolarization phase in nerves. Repolarization (phase 3, point E) in ventricular muscle cells is caused by the opening of a calcium-activated potassium channel. The calcium flowing into the cell during the plateau is responsible for activating this channel.

178–182. The answers are: 178-A, 179-C, 180-D, 181-A, 182-E. *(West, 12/e. pp 239–242.)* The graph accompanying the questions illustrates the development of pressure in the aorta and left atrium and ventricle during the cardiac cycle. A similar set of tracings would be obtained simultaneously from the pulmonary artery and right atrium and ventricle. The magnitude of the pressures attained during systole is lower on the right side. In addition, since pulmonary artery pressure is much lower than aortic pressure, the pulmonic valve opens sooner and right ventricular ejection begins before left ventricular ejection.

During diastole, when the atrioventricular valves are open and the ventricles are filling, atrial and ventricular pressures are identical. Atrial systole or contraction occurring at the end of diastole causes a transient increase in both atrial and ventricular pressures, which ends at point A when the mitral valve closes. Ventricular systole begins with the onset of isovolumetric ventricular contraction (point A). This initial part of systole lasts for 60 ms in the left ventricle and 15 ms in the right ventricle because the right ventricle has to develop less pressure to open the pulmonic valve. During this phase, which ends at point B, both the atrioventricular (mitral) and semilunar (aortic) valves are closed and no further change in ventricular volume occurs. The transient increase in atrial pressure occurring during this interval reflects the bulging of the mitral valve leaflets into the atrium as ventricular pressure rises. With the opening of the aortic valve (point B), ventricular ejection begins. During ventricular ejection, which lasts for 200 ms in the left ventricle and 270 ms in the right ventricle, aortic and left ventricular pressures are nearly identical. Atrial pressure declines initially as the ventricles move away from the atria, but then it gradually rises because of continued atrial filling. As the ventricles begin to relax, both ventricular pressure and aortic pressure fall. When left ventricular pressure falls below aortic pressure (point C), the aortic valve closes. This marks the beginning of isovolumetric ventricular relaxation, which lasts for 100 ms and during which no flow occurs because both the aortic and mitral valves are closed. When ventricular pressure falls below atrial pressure, the mitral valve opens (point D) and ventricular filling (diastole) begins. During the initial filling phase of diastole, both atrial and ventricular pressures decline and ventricular filling is rapid. This is followed by a longer slow filling phase during which atrial and ventricular pressures are the same and gradually rise. This slow filling phase is variable in length; its duration is reduced as heart rate increases.

Depolarization of atria and ventricles precedes the onset of their contraction. The QRS complex of the electrocardiogram is recorded just prior to point A. Ventricular repolarization begins approximately at the midpoint of ventricular ejection and is not identified on the graph.

183–186. The answers are: 183-D, 184-E, 185-B, 186-A. *(Ganong, 15/e. pp 528–531.)* Cardiac output is a function of both stroke volume and heart rate. Alterations in contractility, which influences stroke volume, are termed *inotropic effects*, whereas alterations of rate are termed *chronotropic effects*. The Frank-Starling law of the heart states that the contractility of cardiac muscle is directly related to the initial length of the fiber. Thus, if cardiac muscle fibers are stretched by an increase in end-diastolic volume (acute volume overload), myocardial contractility increases (point D in the graph accompanying the question). In the presence of pericardial effusion, ventricular end-diastolic volume is depressed because of compression and so contractility decreases (point B).

In addition to this autoregulatory mechanism, myocardial contractility also is influenced by metabolic and neural factors. Sympathetic stimulation increases myocardial contractility (positive inotropic effect) and parasympathetic stimulation decreases it (negative inotropic effect). Of these two opposing factors, the sympathetic effect is the more potent and significant. Sympathetic stimulation is mediated by beta-adrenergic receptors. Activation of these receptors results in increased cytoplasmic cyclic AMP, which mediates the inotropic effects. Drugs that inhibit degradation of cyclic AMP, such as caffeine, exert positive inotropic effects. Muscular exercise, by increasing sympathetic discharge, increases contractility as well as venous return (point A).

Hypoxia, hypercapnia, and acidosis all depress myocardial contractility so that for the same ventricular end-diastolic volume, contractility is reduced (point E).

187–190. The answers are: 187-D, 188-C, 189-A, 190-A. *(Ganong, 15/e. pp 550–561.)* Heart rate and blood pressure are regulated by the interaction of the sympathetic and parasympathetic divisions of the autonomic nervous system and medullary centers. Increases in heart rate are generally accompanied by increases in blood pressure. The net effect of both actions is to increase blood flow and improve perfusion.

An increase in intracranial pressure, which compresses cerebral vessels, results in decreased cerebral blood flow. The decrease in flow stimulates both the vasomotor and cardioinhibitory centers, elevating blood pressure and decreasing heart rate.

In exercise, impulses from the cerebral cortex converging on medullary centers as well as direct cardiac sympathetic stimulation result in an increase in blood pressure and tachycardia. During aerobic exercise, total peripheral resistance falls. In extreme cases, this can actually cause a decrease in blood pressure.

In hypoxia, chemoreceptor input into the vasomotor center produces an acceleration of heart rate and an increase in blood pressure. The net effect is improved oxygen delivery to peripheral areas.

Syncope, or fainting, is usually caused by an increase in vagal tone accompanied by a decrease in vasomotor activity. In some cases, the drop in blood pressure stimulates the baroreceptor reflex of the carotid sinus, which causes an increase in heart rate.

Respiratory System

DIRECTIONS: Each question below contains five suggested responses. Select the **one best** response to each question.

191. The basic respiratory rhythm is generated in the

(A) apneustic center
(B) nucleus parabrachialis
(C) dorsal medulla
(D) pneumotaxic center
(E) cerebrum

192. During quiet breathing, at the start of inspiration the intrapleural pressure is about -4 mmHg (relative to atmospheric pressure). As inspiration proceeds, intrapleural pressure reaches approximately

(A) -8 mmHg
(B) -1 mmHg
(C) 0 mmHg
(D) $+1$ mmHg
(E) $+8$ mmHg

193. The bulk of CO_2 is transported in arterial blood as

(A) dissolved CO_2
(B) carbonic acid
(C) carbaminohemoglobin
(D) bicarbonate
(E) carboxyhemoglobin

Questions 194–195

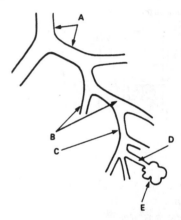

194. In the diagram of a human airway above, gas exchange occurs in

(A) E
(B) E and D
(C) E, D, and C
(D) E, D, C, and B
(E) E, D, C, B, and A

195. In the diagram above, the letter C refers to the

(A) alveolar sac
(B) alveolar duct
(C) respiratory bronchiole
(D) terminal bronchiole
(E) bronchus

196. The oxygen required by the respiratory muscles would be increased by all the following EXCEPT

(A) a decrease in lung compliance
(B) a decrease in airway resistance
(C) an increase in the rate of respiration
(D) a decrease in the production of pulmonary surfactant
(E) an increase in tidal volume

Questions 197–198

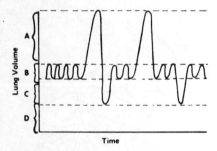

Time

197. In the graph of respiratory excursions shown above, the tidal volume is represented by

(A) A
(B) B
(C) C
(D) D
(E) A plus B

198. The functional residual capacity is represented by

(A) A
(B) B plus C plus D
(C) C
(D) B plus C
(E) C plus D

199. The partial pressure of oxygen in dry air (21% O_2) inhaled by divers at a depth of 100 feet below sea level (4 atmospheres) is approximately

(A) 160 mmHg
(B) 320 mmHg
(C) 640 mmHg
(D) 1280 mmHg
(E) none of the above

200. A patient is on a ventilator adjusted for a tidal volume of 1 L at a frequency of 10/min. If the patient's anatomic dead space is 200 mL and the machine's dead space 50 mL, the alveolar ventilation is

(A) 10 L/min
(B) 8.5 L/min
(C) 7.5 L/min
(D) 5 L/min
(E) not determinable from the information given

201. A person starts to breathe into a 12-L spirometer containing 10% helium at the end of a passive expiration. If, after several minutes, the helium concentration in the spirometer falls to 8%, this person's functional residual capacity (FRC) is approximately

(A) 1 L
(B) 2 L
(C) 3 L
(D) 4 L
(E) 5 L

202. Two healthy women with identical tidal volumes and respiratory rates are subjected to spirometry and blood gas measurements. Subject A doubles her tidal volume and decreases her respiratory rate to one-half of baseline. Subject B decreases her tidal volume to one-half of baseline and doubles her respiratory rate. Which of the following statements about the resulting alveolar ventilation in the two women is true?

(A) Alveolar ventilation is unchanged in both subjects
(B) Alveolar ventilation increases in both subjects
(C) Alveolar ventilation decreases in both subjects
(D) Alveolar ventilation increases in subject A and decreases in subject B
(E) Alveolar ventilation decreases in subject A and increases in subject B

203. The concentration of CO_2 is lowest in

(A) the anatomic dead space at end inspiration
(B) the anatomic dead space at end expiration
(C) the alveoli at end inspiration
(D) the alveoli at end expiration
(E) the blood in the pulmonary veins

204. Functions of alveolar macrophages include all the following EXCEPT

(A) phagocytosis of bacteria
(B) secretion of surfactant
(C) release of lysosomal enzymes into the alveolar space
(D) transport of inhaled particles out of the alveoli
(E) release of leukocyte chemotactic factors

205. Peripheral and central chemoreceptors may both contribute to the increased ventilation that occurs as a result of

(A) a decrease in arterial oxygen content
(B) a decrease in arterial blood pressure
(C) an increase in arterial carbon dioxide tension
(D) a decrease in arterial oxygen tension
(E) an increase in arterial pH

206. Complete transection of the brainstem above the pons would

(A) result in cessation of all breathing movements
(B) prevent any voluntary holding of breath
(C) prevent the central chemoreceptors from exerting any control over ventilation
(D) prevent the peripheral chemoreceptors from exerting any control over ventilation
(E) abolish the Hering-Breuer reflex

Questions 207–208

The diagram below illustrates the change in intrapleural pressure during a single breath.

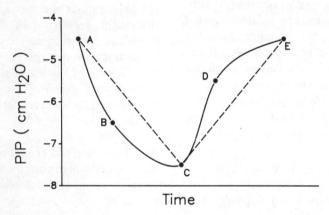

207. At which point on the diagram is inspiratory airflow the greatest?

(A) A
(B) B
(C) C
(D) D
(E) E

208. At which point on the diagram is lung volume the greatest?

(A) A
(B) B
(C) C
(D) D
(E) E

209. The water vapor pressure of alveolar gas at a barometric pressure of 380 mmHg is

(A) 23.5 mmHg
(B) 47.0 mmHg
(C) 76.0 mmHg
(D) 94.0 mmHg
(E) 105.0 mmHg

210. A deficiency of pulmonary surfactant would

(A) decrease surface tension in the alveoli
(B) decrease the change in intra-pleural pressure required to achieve a given tidal volume
(C) decrease lung compliance
(D) decrease the work of breathing
(E) increase functional residual capacity (FRC)

Questions 211–212

Measurement of the closing volume is a sensitive test of airway disease. A patient expires to residual volume and then inspires to total lung volume. At the beginning of this inspiration, a small quantity of insoluble inert tracer gas (helium) is injected into the inspired gas. The patient then expires to residual volume and the curve appearing below is produced.

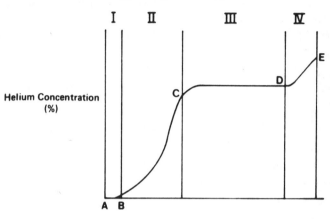

211. Closing volume is measured at point

(A) A
(B) B
(C) C
(D) D
(E) E

212. Closing volume is normally what percentage of vital capacity?

(A) Ten percent in young persons and it increases with age
(B) Ten percent in young persons and it decreases with age
(C) Forty percent in young persons and it increases with age
(D) Forty percent in young persons and it decreases with age
(E) Ninety percent

213. The following data were obtained during a pulmonary function test: fraction of CO_2 in mixed expired gas $(F_E CO_2)$ = 3.0%; fraction of CO_2 in alveolar gas $(F_A CO_2)$ = 4.5%; tidal volume (V_T) = 450 mL (BTPS); and frequency = 10 breaths per minute. The volume of the physiologic dead space (V_D) is

(A) 100 mL
(B) 150 mL
(C) 225 mL
(D) 750 mL
(E) 1500 mL

214. A man breathing at a frequency of 20 breaths per minute has a minute ventilation of 8000 mL/min and a dead space of 150 mL. His alveolar ventilation is

(A) 250 mL/min
(B) 400 mL/min
(C) 2500 mL/min
(D) 3000 mL/min
(E) 5000 mL/min

215. A man breathing room air at sea level has an alveolar ventilation of 2 L/min. The blood gases show a Pa_{CO_2} of 48 mmHg and a Pa_{O_2} of 70 mmHg. The alveolar oxygen tension (PA_{O_2}) is

(A) 150 mmHg
(B) 110 mmHg
(C) 100 mmHg
(D) 90 mmHg
(E) 60 mmHg

216. A young skier with normal pulmonary function (minute volume 4 L; pulmonary blood flow 5 L/min) who is recovering from a tibial fracture suddenly develops right-sided chest pain and tachypnea. Embolic occlusion of the right pulmonary artery is suspected. The diagnosis would be immediately confirmed by which of the following tracheal gas measurements?

	P_{O_2} (mmHg)	P_{CO2} (mmHg)
(A)	125	60
(B)	125	20
(C)	100	40
(D)	80	20
(E)	80	60

217. Measurement of the lecithin-sphingomyelin (L-S) ratio in amniotic fluid assesses

(A) the placenta's ability to oxygenate the fetus
(B) fetal adrenal function
(C) fetal kidney development
(D) fetal brain development
(E) fetal lung maturity

218. When the respiratory muscles are relaxed, the lungs are at

(A) residual volume (RV)
(B) expiratory reserve volume (ERV)
(C) functional residual capacity (FRC)
(D) inspiratory reserve volume (IRV)
(E) total lung capacity (TLC)

219. Which one of the following is the most likely cause of a high arterial P_{CO_2}?

(A) Increased metabolic activity
(B) Increased alveolar dead space
(C) Depressed medullary respiratory centers
(D) Alveolar capillary block
(E) Increased alveolar ventilation

220. The resistance of the large- and medium-sized airways as a percentage of the total airway resistance is approximately

(A) 10 percent
(B) 20 percent
(C) 40 percent
(D) 60 percent
(E) 80 percent

221. Pulmonary vascular resistance increases

(A) as the lung volume approaches TLC
(B) as the lung volume approaches FRC
(C) as the cardiac output increases
(D) as pulmonary artery pressure increases
(E) as left atrial pressure increases

222. Which of the following would normally be found to be less in the fetus than in the mother?

(A) Pa_{CO_2}
(B) Pulmonary vascular resistance
(C) Affinity of hemoglobin for oxygen
(D) Pa_{O_2}
(E) Arterial hydrogen ion concentration ($[H^+]a$)

223. During a forced expiration, actively contracting muscles include the

(A) sternocleidomastoid
(B) diaphragm
(C) abdominal muscles
(D) external intercostals
(E) scalene

224. During moderate aerobic exercise,

(A) Pa_{O_2} increases
(B) Pa_{CO_2} decreases
(C) arterial pH decreases
(D) alveolar ventilation increases
(E) blood lactate level increases

225. Reduction of functional hemoglobin associated with anemia, methemoglobinemia, or carbon monoxide poisoning does not produce hyperpnea because the

(A) blood flow to the carotid body is decreased
(B) total arterial oxygen content is maintained within the normal range
(C) carotid body chemoreceptors are stimulated
(D) central chemoreceptors are stimulated
(E) P_{O_2} of arterial blood is normal

226. Characteristics of blood in the pulmonary circulation include all the following EXCEPT

(A) volume of about 1 L
(B) flow rate of about 5.5 L/min
(C) volume in the capillaries of less than 100 mL
(D) flow rate that increases during exercise
(E) flow that is nonpulsatile

227. Pulmonary alveoli are kept dry by factors that include the

(A) phagocytic activity of alveolar macrophages
(B) negative interstitial fluid pressure
(C) low vapor pressure of water in inspired air
(D) secretion of surfactant
(E) tight junctions between the alveolar capillary endothelial cells

228. All the following are characteristics of the lung EXCEPT

(A) the interstitial colloid oncotic pressure is about 15 mmHg
(B) filtration is continuous along the length of the alveolar capillary
(C) the hydrostatic pressure in the pulmonary capillaries is the same as in the systemic capillaries
(D) filtered H_2O is removed by the lymphatics
(E) the interstitial hydrostatic pressure is subatmospheric

229. In a normal, standing person, all the following will contribute significantly to the existence of the alveolar-arterial (A-a) gradient for O_2 EXCEPT

(A) variations in the V/Q ratios throughout the lungs
(B) a small right-to-left absolute shunt
(C) the nonlinearity of the oxyhemoglobin dissociation curve
(D) the disequilibrium of end-pulmonary capillary P_{O_2} and alveolar P_{O_2}
(E) blood flow from the bronchial circulation

230. Surfactant is accurately described by all the following statements EXCEPT

(A) it is a lipoprotein containing dipalmitoyl lecithin
(B) it is responsible for the hysteresis demonstrated in the pressure-volume curve characteristic of the human lung
(C) it reduces surface tension in the alveoli
(D) it is made in type II cells
(E) it is present in increased amounts in hyaline membrane disease

231. As the P_{CO_2} of the venous blood increases,

(A) the concentration of HCO_3^- decreases
(B) the concentration of H^+ in the red cell decreases
(C) the volume of the red cell increases
(D) the affinity of the hemoglobin for O_2 increases
(E) the amount of chloride in the red cell decreases

232. Metabolic functions of the lung include all the following EXCEPT

(A) inactivation of angiotensin II
(B) inactivation of bradykinin
(C) inactivation of prostaglandins
(D) synthesis of prostaglandins
(E) synthesis of surfactant

233. Factors in determining the diffusion capacity of the lung for oxygen (D_LO_2) include all the following EXCEPT

(A) the cardiac output
(B) the oxygen partial pressure gradient from alveolar gas to pulmonary capillary blood
(C) the concentration of hemoglobin in the pulmonary capillary blood
(D) the alveolar surface area
(E) the thickness of the alveolar-capillary membrane

234. Venous admixture is produced by blood from all the following EXCEPT

(A) the thebesian veins
(B) high V/Q areas of the lung
(C) the bronchial veins
(D) right-to-left intracardiac shunts
(E) alveoli with impaired diffusion

235. The percentage of hemoglobin saturated with oxygen will increase if

(A) the arterial P_{CO_2} is increased
(B) the hemoglobin concentration is increased
(C) the temperature is increased
(D) the arterial P_{O_2} is increased
(E) the arterial pH is decreased

236. Which of the following will return toward normal during acclimatization to high altitude?

(A) Arterial hydrogen ion concentration
(B) Arterial carbon dioxide tension
(C) Arterial bicarbonate ion concentration
(D) Arterial hemoglobin concentration
(E) Alveolar ventilation

237. In a normal person, end-pulmonary capillary blood would reach diffusional equilibrium with the alveolar partial pressure of all the following EXCEPT

(A) oxygen
(B) nitrogen
(C) carbon dioxide
(D) carbon monoxide
(E) nitrous oxide (N_2O)

238. Shift of the CO_2 response curve from curve A to curve B as shown below would be produced by all the following EXCEPT

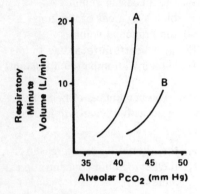

(A) diazepam
(B) barbiturates
(C) morphine
(D) sleep
(E) exercise

239. Pulmonary compliance is characterized by which of the following statements?

(A) It decreases with advancing age
(B) It is inversely related to the elastic recoil properties of the lung
(C) It increases in patients with pulmonary edema
(D) It is equivalent to $\Delta P/\Delta V$
(E) It increases when there is a deficiency of surfactant

240. The activity of the central chemoreceptors is stimulated by

(A) an increase in the P_{CO_2} of blood flowing through the brain
(B) a decrease in the P_{O_2} of blood flowing through the brain
(C) a decrease in the oxygen content of blood flowing through the brain
(D) a decrease in the metabolic rate of the surrounding brain tissue
(E) an increase in the pH of the CSF

241. Hypoxemia (Pa_{O_2} = 55 mmHG) has all the following effects EXCEPT

(A) it stimulates carotid body chemoreceptors
(B) it stimulates central chemoreceptors
(C) it stimulates aortic body chemoreceptors
(D) it causes a reflex increase in ventilation
(E) it causes a reflex increase in arterial blood pressure

242. In an acclimatized person at high altitudes, oxygen delivery to the tissues may be adequate at rest because of

(A) an increase in hemoglobin concentration
(B) the presence of an acidosis
(C) a decrease in the number of tissue capillaries
(D) the presence of a normal arterial P_{O_2}
(E) the presence of a lower-than-normal arterial P_{CO_2}

243. Which of the following will increase as a result of stimulating parasympathetic nerves to the bronchial smooth muscle?

(A) Lung compliance
(B) Airway diameter
(C) Elastic work of breathing
(D) Resistive work of breathing
(E) Anatomic dead space

244. Hyperventilation may be produced by stimulation of all the following receptors EXCEPT

(A) peripheral chemoreceptors
(B) irritant receptors
(C) peripheral pain receptors
(D) pulmonary stretch receptors
(E) J (juxtacapillary) receptors

245. During a normal inspiration, more air goes to the alveoli at the base of the lung than to the alveoli at the apex of the lung because

(A) the alveoli at the base of the lung have more surfactant
(B) the alveoli at the base of the lung are more compliant
(C) the alveoli at the base of the lung have higher V/Q ratios
(D) there is a more negative intrapleural pressure at the base of the lung
(E) there is more blood flow to the base of the lung

246. A pulmonary arterial (Swan-Ganz) catheter can be used for all the following EXCEPT

(A) to measure pulmonary artery diastolic pressure
(B) to measure pulmonary artery systolic pressure
(C) to measure pulmonary capillary wedge pressure
(D) to estimate aortic pressure
(E) to estimate left atrial pressure

247. A spirometer can be used to measure directly

(A) functional residual capacity
(B) inspiratory capacity
(C) residual volume
(D) total lung capacity
(E) none of the above

DIRECTIONS: Each group of questions below consists of lettered headings followed by a set of numbered items. For each numbered item select the **one** lettered heading with which it is **most** closely associated. Each lettered heading may be used **once, more than once, or not at all.**

Questions 248–255

For each situation described below, select the combination of arterial blood pH and P_{CO_2} with which it is most likely to be associated.

(A) Increased pH, increased P_{CO_2}
(B) Increased pH, decreased P_{CO_2}
(C) Decreased pH, decreased P_{CO_2}
(D) Decreased pH, increased P_{CO_2}
(E) Normal pH, decreased P_{CO_2}

248. Suddenly increased respiratory rate, unchanged tidal volume

249. Increased tidal volume, unchanged respiratory rate

250. Living at a high altitude

251. Anxiety-induced hyperventilation

252. Diabetic acidosis

253. Respiratory arrest

254. Administration of CO_2

255. Metabolic alkalosis

Questions 256–264

For blood under each of the conditions described below, select the oxyhemoglobin dissociation curve with which it is most likely to be associated.

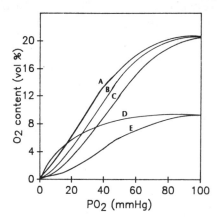

256. Blood with a Pa_{CO_2} above normal

257. Normal adult arterial blood

258. Fetal blood

259. Blood stored for 3 weeks

260. Anemic blood

261. Blood with a pHa above normal

262. Blood from a patient with hypothermia

263. Blood with an increased level of 2,3-diphosphoglycerate (2,3-DPG)

264. Blood exposed to carbon monoxide

DIRECTIONS: Each group of questions below consists of four lettered headings followed by a set of numbered items. For each numbered item select

A	if the item is associated with	**A only**
B	if the item is associated with	**(B) only**
C	if the item is associated with	**both** (A) and (B)
D	if the item is associated with	**neither** (A) nor (B)

Each lettered heading may be used **once, more than once, or not at all.**

Questions 265–267

(A) A lower-than-normal Pa_{O_2}
(B) A lower-than-normal Pa_{CO_2}
(C) Both
(D) Neither

265. End-pulmonary capillary blood from areas of the lung that have low V/Q ratios

266. End-pulmonary capillary blood from areas of the lung that have high V/Q ratios

267. Arterial blood from a patient with a blocked right main bronchus

Questions 268–269

(A) Concentration of hemoglobin
(B) Alveolar P_{O_2}
(C) Both
(D) Neither

268. Will determine the oxygen content of the end-pulmonary capillary blood in a normal person

269. Will determine the percentage of hemoglobin saturated with oxygen in the end-pulmonary capillary blood of a normal person

Questions 270–278

(A) Restrictive lung disease
(B) Obstructive lung disease
(C) Both
(D) Neither

270. Asthma

271. Respiratory distress syndrome in the infant

272. Lung fibrosis

273. Decreased lung compliance

274. Rapid, shallow breathing

275. Slow, deep breathing

276. Decreased functional residual capacity (FRC)

277. Decreased forced expiratory volume expelled in 1 s (FEV_1)

278. Decreased FEV_1/VC

Respiratory System

Answers

191. The answer is C. *(West, 12/e. pp 579–580.)* The basic respiratory rhythm originates from spontaneous rhythmic discharge of inspiratory neurons located in the respiratory center in the dorsal medulla. This basic rhythm can be modified by many factors, including voluntary control of breathing. In the pons are the apneustic center and the pneumotaxic center (which is located in the nucleus parabrachialis). These modify and regularize the basic respiratory rhythm to produce adequate breathing.

192. The answer is A. *(West, 12/e. pp 569–570.)* Because of the presence of elastic tissue in the lung and because of the surface tension of the alveolar lining, the lungs tend to collapse and recoil away from the chest wall. However, the intrapleural, or recoil, pressure prevents collapse. During inspiration, expansion of the thoracic cage stretches the lungs and increases the tendency for the lungs to collapse, a tendency that is opposed by a further decrease in intrapleural pressure.

193. The answer is D. *(Berne, 2/e. pp 613–614.)* CO_2 is transported in arterial blood in three forms: as physically dissolved CO_2 (about 5 percent), in combination with the amino groups of hemoglobin as carbaminohemoglobin (about 5 percent), and as bicarbonate ion HCO_3^- (about 90 percent). The amount of CO_2 actually carried as carbonic acid (H_2CO_3) is negligible. Carboxyhemoglobin refers to the combination of carbon monoxide (CO) and hemoglobin.

194–195. The answers are: 194-C, 195-C. *(West, 12/e. pp 518–520.)* In humans, the airway begins with the trachea and major bronchi and terminates in the alveolar sacs. The trachea and bronchi (A in the diagram accompanying the question) are lined by ciliated columnar epithelium with numerous mucous glands that provide lubrication and cleansing action. The distal airway includes the terminal bronchiole (B), respiratory bronchiole (C), alveolar duct (D), and alveolar sacs (E). The surface distal to the terminal bronchiole is covered by a thin epithelial lining that is separated from the interstitium and capillary wall by a thin basement membrane. This "respiratory membrane" has an overall thickness ranging from 0.2 to 0.5 μ. It is across this surface that CO_2 and O_2 exchange occurs by passive diffusion. In adults, the total surface area across which this exchange occurs is approximately 70 m². Because total pulmonary capillary blood volume is approximately 100 mL, gas exchange is rapid.

196. The answer is B. *(West, 12/e. pp 577–578.)* Respiratory muscles consume oxygen in proportion to the work of breathing, which can be divided into resistance work and compliance, or elastic, work. Resistance work includes work to overcome tissue as well as airway resistance. A decrease in the amount of pulmonary surfactant would decrease lung compliance and increase the elastic work of breathing. An increase in respiratory rate would increase both types of the work of breathing.

197–198. The answers are: 197-B, 198-E. *(West, 12/e. pp 522–524.)* In respiration, tidal volume is the volume of each normal breath and would be designated by interval B in the graph accompanying the questions. Tidal volume ranges from 400 to 500 mL in the normal adult.

Inspiratory capacity (interval A plus B), which is the maximum volume that can be inspired beginning at the end of normal expiration, averages about 3600 mL. Additional air that can be expired from the resting end-expiratory level, termed *expiratory reserve* (interval C), is about 1000 mL. The lungs do not, however, become airless if expiratory reserve is expelled. The remaining volume, which cannot be removed by forced expiration, is termed *residual volume* (interval D). This residual volume reduces the work required to reexpand the lungs during the next cycle.

The total volume of air remaining at the resting end-expiratory position is the functional residual capacity (FRC). This FRC (interval C plus D) prevents extreme changes in P_{O_2} that would occur during ventilation if the entire alveolar volume were replaced.

The respiratory relationships described above are illustrated in the following graph:

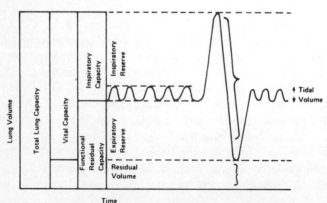

199. The answer is C. *(West, 12/e. p 521.)* According to Dalton's law of partial pressures, each component in a gas mixture exerts a pressure proportional to its concentration in the mixture, and the sum of the pressures of the components is equal to the total pressure of the gas. In air at 4 atmospheres (4 × 760 mmHg) the partial pressure of oxygen would be $0.21 \times 4 \times 760 = 640$ mmHg. Long-term exposure to such an elevated P_{O_2} can have harmful effects on both pulmonary and neural function.

200. The answer is C. *(West, 12/e. pp 524–525.)* Total ventilation is simply tidal volume times frequency. Some of this, however, is wasted ventilation of dead space. In the example provided in the question, the patient's and the machine's dead spaces must be added to determine the total dead space in each breath (of 1 L); the remainder is the alveolar ventilation. Thus, alveolar ventilation = $(1000 \text{ mL} - 200 \text{ mL} - 50 \text{ mL}) \times 10/\text{min} = 7.5$ L/min.

201. The answer is C. *(Berne, 2/e. pp 594–595. West, 12/e. pp 523–524.)* The helium dilution method can be used to determine FRC (which equals RV + ERV) since RV cannot be determined directly by spirometry. This method relies on the conservation of mass. A known volume and concentration (amount) of helium (which is inert in the body) is diluted by an unknown volume (the FRC of the person). The resulting helium concentration is measured, and since the amount of helium remains the same, the added volume—the FRC—can be calculated:

$$\text{Spirometer vol.} \times \text{initial \%He} = (\text{FRC} + \text{spirometer vol.}) \times \text{final \%He}$$
$$12 \text{ L} \times 10\% = (\text{FRC} + 12) \times 8\%$$
$$\text{FRC} = 3 \text{ L}$$

202. The answer is D. *(West, 12/e. pp 523–527.)* Changes in tidal volume (TV) have a greater effect on alveolar ventilation ($\dot{V}_A$) than do equivalent changes in respiratory rate (RR) because of the contribution of the dead space. This relationship can be seen from the expression

$$\dot{V}_A = \text{RR (TV − dead space)}$$

Assuming, for example, that TV = 500 mL, RR = 12/min, and dead space = 150 mL,

$$\dot{V}_A = 12 (500 - 150) = 4200 \text{ mL/min}$$

If TV is doubled and RR halved,

$$TV \times 2 = 1000 \text{ mL}$$
$$RR \div 2 = 6/\text{min}$$
$$\text{and } \dot{V}_A = 6 (1000 - 150) = 5100 \text{ mL/min}$$

But if TV is halved and RR doubled,

$$TV \div 2 = 250 \text{ mL}$$
$$RR \times 2 = 24/\text{min}$$
$$\text{and } \dot{V}_A = 24 (250 - 150) = 2400 \text{ mL/min}$$

203. The answer is A. *(Guyton, 8/e. pp 424–426.)* The anatomic dead space, which includes the trachea, bronchi, and bronchioles, is filled with fresh room air at the end of an inspiration and with end-expired, or alveolar, gas at the end of an expiration. Room air contains very little CO_2 (0.03 percent), whereas alveolar air contains considerably more CO_2 (about 5.5 percent) as a result of gas exchange in the lungs. The P_{CO_2} of alveolar air does fluctuate to some extent with each breath because it is diluted with fresh air during inspiration. The P_{CO_2} of the blood in the pulmonary veins is in equilibrium with that in the alveoli.

204. The answer is B. *(Ganong, 15/e. pp 614–615. West, 12/e. pp 345–346.)* Alveolar macrophages are cells that migrate over the alveolar epithelial surface within the surfactant layer. They are phagocytic cells and ingest inhaled bacteria and particulate matter. This phagocytic activity is often associated with release of leukocyte chemotactic factors and lysosomal enzymes into the extracellular space, which can result in damage to normal tissue by eliciting the inflammatory reaction. Undigested particulate matter is transported out of alveoli by either being carried up the bronchial tree by ciliary action or by circulation through interstitial lymphatic channels. Though macrophages often contain ingested surfactant material, they have not been shown to synthesize surfactant, a product of alveolar type II epithelial cells.

205. The answer is C. *(West, 12/e. pp 580–582, 583–585.)* The central chemoreceptors located on or near the ventral surface of the medulla cause an increase in ventilation in response to an increase in Pa_{CO_2} and to a lesser extent to a decrease in arterial pH because the blood-brain barrier is relatively impermeable to hydrogen ions. The peripheral chemoreceptors in the carotid bodies cause an increase in ventilation in response to an increase in Pa_{CO_2}, a decrease in arterial pH, and a decrease in Pa_{O_2}. Neither the central chemoreceptors nor the carotid bodies are stimulated by a decrease in arterial blood pressure or O_2 content.

206. The answer is B. *(Ganong, 15/e. pp 623–631.)* Transection of the brainstem above the pons would prevent any voluntary changes in ventilation by cutting the pathways from the higher centers. Breathing would continue because the pontine-medullary centers that control rhythmic ventilation would be intact. Inputs to the brainstem from the central and peripheral chemoreceptors that stimulate ventilation and from lung stretch receptors that inhibit inspiration (Hering-Breuer reflex) would also be intact and these reflexes would be maintained.

207–208. The answers are: 207-B, 208-C. *(West, 12/e. pp 569–570.)* During inspiration (curve ABC) the respiratory muscles pull the chest wall out and diaphragm down and intrapleural pressure (P_{IP}) becomes more negative. The muscles must overcome the elastic recoil forces of the lungs and the resistance of the airways to airflow. The P_{IP} necessary to overcome the elastic forces of the lung is depicted by dashed line AC. The P_{IP} necessary to overcome the airway resistance is the difference between dashed line AC and curve ABC. The maximum airflow occurs at point B, where the difference between the two is the greatest. Lung volume is the greatest at point C, where P_{IP} is the most negative.

209. The answer is B. *(Berne, 2/e. p 605. West, 12/e. p 521.)* Water vapor pressure is independent of the barometric pressure and depends only on the temperature of a gas and the percentage of saturation. By the time inspired gas reaches the alveoli it is at body temperature (37°C) and fully saturated with water. Water vapor pressure of saturated gas at 37°C is 47 mmHg.

210. The answer is C. *(West, 12/e. pp 561–566.)* Because of the inherent elasticity of the lung, the alveoli tend to collapse during expiration. This tendency is explained by Laplace's law, which relates the radius (R) and surface tension (T) of an elastic bubble to the pressure (P) required to distend it, as follows: $P = 2T \div R$. If T were constant, the pressure required to distend alveoli would increase markedly during expiration as the radius decreased. This does not occur in normal lungs because the unique properties of surfactant result in reduced surface tension as the alveolar lining is compressed with the decrease in the alveolar radius during expiration. Thus, surfactant prevents alveolar collapse at end-expiratory intraalveolar pressures that otherwise would lead to atelectasis. A deficiency of surfactant would therefore increase surface tension, tending to collapse the lungs and decrease FRC. It would be more difficult to expand the lungs. Lung compliance would decrease, and thus

a greater change in intrapleural pressure and greater work to maintain ventilation would be required.

211–212. The answers are: 211-D, 212-A. *(West, 12/e. pp 575–576.)* In the
diagram accompanying the question, zones I through IV represent gas from
different topographical areas of the lung. Zone I represents dead space, zone
II is a mixture of dead space and alveolar gas, and zone III represents pure
alveolar gas. At point D the tracer content of expired gas increases. That point
represents the closing volume, which is the lung volume at which airways in
the lower parts of the lung close off because the transmural pressure gradient
is lower owing to the effects of gravity. The gas in the apices (zone IV) is
richer in the tracer gas because the alveoli in that portion of the lung receive
more gas during the early part of inspiration. The closing volume represents
approximately 10 percent of vital capacity and increases with age, as does
residual volume.

213. The answer is B. *(Berne, 2/e. pp 606–607. West, 12/e. pp 527, 559.)* The
volume of the physiologic dead space (V_D) can be calculated using the Bohr
equation:

$$V_D = \left(\frac{F_A CO_2 - F_E CO_2}{F_A CO_2} \right) V_T$$

V_T is tidal volume, $F_A CO_2$ is the fraction of CO_2 in alveolar gas, and $F_E CO_2$ is
the fraction of CO_2 in mixed expired gas. $F_A CO_2$ can be approximated using
the FCO_2 from a sample of end-expiratory gas or by sampling Pa_{CO_2}. In normal
lungs, physiologic dead space equals anatomic dead space. In diseased lungs,
physiologic dead space often exceeds anatomic dead space because of abnormalities of ventilation and blood flow.

214. The answer is E. *(West, 12/e. pp 524–525.)* Minute volume, or minute
ventilation, is the tidal volume times the breathing frequency. This includes
both alveolar ventilation ($\dot{V}_A$) and dead space ventilation ($\dot{V}_D$): minute ventilation = $\dot{V}_A + \dot{V}_D$. Dead space ventilation is the dead space volume (V_D)
times the breathing frequency (f): $\dot{V}_D = V_D \times f$. Substitution into the equations yields

$$8000 \text{ mL/min} = \dot{V}_A + 150 \text{ mL (20 breaths per minute)}$$
$$\dot{V}_A = 5000 \text{ mL/min}$$

215. The answer is D. *(West, 12/e. pp 546–548, 559.)* In patients, it is useful
to calculate the alveolar oxygen tension (PA_{O_2}) in order to assess the alveolar-

arterial oxygen gradient. $P_{A_{O_2}}$ can be calculated using the alveolar gas equation:

$$P_{A_{O_2}} = P_{I_{O_2}} - P_{A_{CO_2}} \left(F_{I_{O_2}} + \frac{1 - F_{I_{O_2}}}{R} \right)$$

This equation can be greatly simplified without sacrificing a great deal of accuracy. The modified alveolar gas equation is

$$P_{A_{O_2}} = P_{I_{O_2}} - \frac{P_{A_{CO_2}}}{R}$$

$P_{A_{CO_2}}$ is equivalent to Pa_{CO_2}. R is the respiratory exchange ratio ($\dot{V}CO_2/\dot{V}O_2$), which depends on the diet and is normally 0.8. $P_{I_{O_2}}$ equals the fraction of oxygen in room air (0.21) times the barometric pressure at sea level (760 mmHg) minus the water vapor pressure (47 mmHg) of saturated tracheal gas at body temperature (37°C):

$$\begin{aligned} P_{A_{O_2}} &= 0.21 \,(760 \text{ mmHg} - 47 \text{ mmHg}) - \frac{48 \text{ mmHg}}{0.8} \\ &= 150 \text{ mmHg} - 60 \text{ mmHg} \\ &= 90 \text{ mmHg} \end{aligned}$$

216. The answer is B. *(West, 12/e. pp 554–558.)* Under normal conditions the V/Q ratio in both lungs is the same, so that mixed alveolar gas in the trachea has the same P_{O_2} and P_{CO_2} as arterial blood (P_{O_2} = 100 mmHg, P_{CO_2} = 40 mmHg). Immediately following complete occlusion of one pulmonary artery, however, equal ventilation of both lungs continues, but all blood flow is directed to one lung. Equal volumes of gas will continue to mix in the trachea, but the gas from the occluded lung, which now represents alveolar dead space, will be unchanged from room air (P_{O_2} = 150 mmHg, P_{CO_2} = 0.3 mmHg); and gas from the functioning lung will still be normal (P_{O_2} = 100 mmHg, P_{CO_2} = 40 mmHg). Since equal volumes of gas mix, P_{O_2} in the trachea will be (150 + 100) ÷ 2, or 125 mmHg, and P_{CO_2} will be (40 + 0.3) ÷ 2, or 20 mmHg. Such values could occur in normal lungs following hyperventilation but would be accompanied by changes in arterial P_{CO_2}.

217. The answer is E. *(Ganong, 15/e. pp 606–607.)* Lecithin (phosphatidylcholine) and sphingomyelin are choline phospholipids found in a variety of tissues. Lecithin is a major component of surfactant and its synthesis increases as the fetus matures and the lungs are prepared for expansion. Surfactant, a lipoprotein mixture, prevents alveolar collapse by permitting the surface tension of the alveolar lining to vary during inspiration and expiration. Thus, measurement of the lecithin-sphingomyelin (L-S) ratio in amniotic fluid provides an index of fetal lung maturity.

218. The answer is C. *(Berne, 2/e. pp 580–584.)* The lungs tend to recoil inward, whereas the chest wall tends to recoil outward. When the respiratory muscles are all relaxed, these two opposing forces are balanced. The volume of gas in the lungs at this point is the relaxation volume, or functional residual capacity (FRC).

219. The answer is C. *(Berne, 2/e. pp 607–609, 627–629, 637–638. West, 12/e. pp 546–548, 558.)* A high arterial P_{CO_2} is most likely caused by depressed medullary respiratory centers. Depression of these centers decreases alveolar ventilation and results in hypoventilation with an increased Pa_{CO_2} and decreased Pa_{O_2}. This depression can be caused by drugs such as barbiturates or narcotics. Slight depression also occurs during sleep. If metabolic activity increases, as during mild exercise, alveolar ventilation increases in parallel and Pa_{CO_2} does not change. Retention of CO_2 could result from alveolar capillary block, but it would have to be extremely severe because CO_2 is so soluble in tissue.

220. The answer is E. *(West, 12/e. pp 568–572.)* Although it may seem paradoxical, about 80 percent of the total resistance to airflow occurs in the large- and medium-sized airways. Turbulent flow, which increases the pressure necessary to cause gas to flow, is more likely to occur in larger airways. In patients, an increased resistance to airflow usually indicates the presence of disease of the large airways.

221. The answer is A. *(West, 12/e. pp 530–532.)* Pulmonary vascular resistance changes as lung volume changes. At TLC, expansion of the alveoli increases the pulmonary vascular resistance by compressing the alveolar capillaries. At RV, there is compression of the extraalveolar vessels, which increases the pulmonary vascular resistance. At FRC, the compression by either mechanism is minimal. Pulmonary vascular resistance decreases as left atrial pressure increases, as cardiac output increases, or as pulmonary artery pressure increases because of recruitment and distention of pulmonary capillaries.

222. The answer is D. *(Ganong, 15/e. pp 492–493, 532. West, 12/e. pp 898–900.)* Because fetal hemoglobin (hemoglobin F) is chemically different from adult hemoglobin in that it has two α and two γ chains instead of two α and two β chains, it has a greater affinity for oxygen. This is advantageous in the placental exchange of O_2 from maternal blood (Pa_{O_2} = 100 mmHg) to fetal blood (Pa_{O_2} = 25 mmHg). Pa_{CO_2} is about 2 to 3 mmHg higher in the fetus than in the mother. [H^+]a is about the same in both. Pulmonary vascular resistance is high in the fetus, shunting blood away from the lungs. It decreases at birth and remains low.

223. The answer is C. *(Berne, 2/e. pp 577–579.)* Expiration is normally a passive process that does not require the involvement of any muscles. In a forced expiration the internal intercostal muscles contract, pulling the rib cage downward. The abdominal muscles also contract, which increases intraabdominal pressure and pulls the rib cage downward and inward. The diaphragm and external intercostal muscles contract during inspiration. The scalene and sternocleidomastoid muscles, which assist in expanding the chest wall in inspiration, are important accessory muscles of respiration.

224. The answer is D. *(Berne, 2/e. p 638. Ganong, 15/e. pp 632–633.)* During moderate aerobic exercise, oxygen consumption and CO_2 production increase, but alveolar ventilation increases in parallel. Thus, Pa_{O_2} and Pa_{CO_2} do not change. Arterial pH does not decrease and blood lactate concentration does not increase during moderate aerobic exercise, but arterial pH does decrease and blood lactate concentration does increase during anaerobic exercise because of increased production of lactic acid.

225. The answer is E. *(Ganong, 15/e. pp 625–628.)* The reduction in functional hemoglobin that occurs in anemia, methemoglobinemia, or carboxyhemoglobinemia lessens the total oxygen *content* (dissolved O_2 + HbO_2) in the blood but not the oxygen *tension* (P_{O_2}). Because the chemoreceptors of the carotid body are sensitive to the P_{O_2} of arterial blood and blood flow to the carotid body is normally very high, under conditions in which dissolved oxygen and P_{O_2} are normal the amount of O_2 delivered per unit time is sufficient to prevent activation of the chemoreceptors and no hyperpnea ensues. Central chemoreceptors are stimulated by decreases in the pH of brain extracellular fluid. They do not respond to changes in P_{O_2}.

226. The answer is E. *(Ganong, 15/e. pp 611–614.)* The rate of pulmonary blood flow, or the amount of blood entering the lungs per minute, equals the cardiac output. Normally, the lung contains about 1 L of blood, or one-fifth of the total blood volume. Of this, less than 100 mL are contained in capillaries, where most gas exchange occurs. A red blood cell traverses the pulmonary capillaries in about 0.75 s when the body is at rest. During exercise, this time interval may fall to 0.3 s or less, and the rate of pulmonary blood flow may increase to 40 L/min. Blood flow in the pulmonary capillaries is pulsatile.

227. The answer is B. *(West, 12/e. pp 535–536.)* The forces tending to remove fluid from the alveoli are the negative interstitial fluid pressure and the osmotic pressure exerted at the alveolar membrane by ions and crystalloid molecules in the interstitial fluid. Fluid movement into pulmonary *capillaries*, however, is a function of plasma *oncotic* pressure. The pulmonary capillaries are actually leakier than those in the systemic circulation; i.e., they have a higher hydraulic conductivity. Alveolar phagocytes do not take up significant amounts of water, and very little water from the alveoli goes into inspired air because the air is well humidified by the upper airways. Surfactant lowers the surface tension in the alveoli but does not affect fluid movement.

228. The answer is C. *(Berne, 2/e. pp 602–603.)* The pulmonary circulation is a low-pressure system. Thus the hydrostatic pressure in the pulmonary capillaries is about 10 mmHg and is less than in the systemic capillaries. It is greater at the base of the lung than at the apex because of increased hydrostatic pressure at the base. The colloid osmotic pressure in the pulmonary capillary is about 25 mmHg and that in the interstitial space is estimated to be about 15 mmHg. The interstitial hydrostatic pressure is estimated to be slightly negative. Thus the balance of these Starling forces favors continuous filtration out of the capillaries into the interstitial space. This continuous flow of fluid is removed by the very efficient lymphatic system in the lungs.

229. The answer is D. *(Berne, 2/e. pp 615–619. West, 12/e. pp 553–559.)* In a normal person there is an A-a gradient for O_2 of about 4 to 10 mmHg. The V/Q ratios at the apices of the lungs are greater than at the bases of the lungs; this results in end-pulmonary capillary blood coming from the apices with higher P_{O_2} and from the bases with lower P_{O_2} than normal. The P_{O_2} of the mixed blood from these areas must be determined by the average of their O_2 contents. Because of the nonlinearity of the oxyhemoglobin dissociation curve, the resultant Pa_{O_2} is not the average of the end-pulmonary capillary P_{O_2} values. In addition, about 2 to 5 percent of the blood returning to the left heart—i.e., blood from the bronchial veins and from the thebesian veins draining the left ventricle—is venous blood that has not been oxygenated and constitutes a right-to-left absolute shunt. Normally levels of alveolar and end-pulmonary capillary blood P_{O_2} do come into equilibrium. If they do not, as in some disease states, this alveolar-capillary block would contribute to the A-a gradient for O_2.

230. The answer is E. *(West, 12/e. pp 564–566.)* Surfactant is a lipoprotein mixture rich in dipalmitoyl lecithin, which is made by type II pneumonocytes lining the alveoli. It acts to diminish surface tension when alveolar volume decreases so that the pressure required to maintain the smaller alveolar volume is decreased, thus averting alveolar collapse at zero pressure. Because reexpansion requires sufficient pressure to overcome both surface tension and tissue elasticity, the pressure-volume curves for inflation and deflation do not coincide, and hysteresis results. Hyaline membrane disease (respiratory distress syndrome) results from a deficiency of surfactant and is accompanied by atelectasis.

231. The answer is C. *(Berne, 2/e. pp 613–615. West, 12/e. pp 540–542.)* In the tissues, CO_2 diffuses into the blood down its concentration gradient. CO_2 enters the red cells where carbonic anhydrase accelerates its hydration reaction.

$$CO_2 + H_2O \stackrel{CA}{\rightleftharpoons} H_2CO_3 \rightleftharpoons H^+ + HCO_3^-$$

Thus, the concentrations of H^+ and HCO_3^- in the red cell rise. Most of the H^+ is buffered by hemoglobin, but the new HCO_3^- ion constitutes a new osmotic particle in the red cell and the red cell swells. Most of the HCO_3^- exchanges for Cl^- across the red cell membrane, which increases the amount of the chloride in the red cell. The increased P_{CO_2} and concentration of H^+ cause a decrease in the affinity of hemoglobin for O_2.

232. The answer is A. *(West, 12/e. pp 536–537.)* The lung has many metabolic functions, including synthesis of surfactant and prostaglandins and withdrawal of prostaglandins and bradykinin from the circulation. Other metabolic functions include activation of angiotensin I to angiotensin II, release of histamine, and inactivation of serotonin. Prostaglandins E and F both are synthesized and removed from the circulation by the lungs.

233. The answer is B. *(Berne, 2/e. pp 622–623. West, 12/e. pp 550–552.)* The diffusing capacity of the lung for oxygen (D_LO_2) is the amount of oxygen that crosses the alveolar-capillary membranes per minute per millimeter of mercury of partial pressure difference between the alveolar gas and the pulmonary capillary blood. A normal resting value is about 25 mL/min/mmHg. D_LO_2 depends on the area available for gas exchange, which includes the number of open capillaries in the lung and the thickness of the alveolar-capillary membrane. When cardiac output increases (e.g., during exercise), D_LO_2 increases because more pulmonary capillaries open up. D_LO_2 also depends on the amount of hemoglobin present to take up oxygen in the pulmonary capillary blood.

234. The answer is B. *(West, 12/e. pp 553–556.)* Venous admixture is the addition of blood with a lower P_{O_2} to oxygenated blood returning to the left side of the heart. In a normal person, this lowers the arterial P_{O_2} by about 5 mmHg. This blood includes flow from the thebesian veins, which drain the myocardium of the left ventricle; from the bronchial veins, which drain the walls of the airways; from areas of the lung with lower-than-normal V/Q ratios; and from alveoli with impaired diffusion, if any are present. Venous admixture is also referred to as *right-to-left shunt flow*.

235. The answer is D. *(Berne, 2/e. pp 609–612.)* The percentage of hemoglobin saturated with oxygen depends on the level of P_{O_2} in the blood and on other factors that affect the position of the oxyhemoglobin dissociation curve. Factors that shift the curve to the left, such as a decrease in P_{CO_2}, an increase in pH, or a decrease in temperature, would increase the percentage of hemoglobin saturated with oxygen as would an increase in P_{O_2} provided that the percentage of saturation was not already at 100 percent. At a given P_{O_2}, increasing the concentration of hemoglobin would not affect the percentage of saturation but would increase the oxygen content of blood.

236. The answer is A. *(West, 12/e. pp 588–592.)* At high altitude, the barometric pressure is reduced, resulting in a decrease in $P_{I_{O_2}}$, which decreases both alveolar and arterial P_{O_2}. If Pa_{O_2} is less than 60 mmHg, the carotid bodies are stimulated and cause hyperventilation, which increases alveolar ventilation and decreases Pa_{CO_2} with a resultant respiratory alkalosis. During acclimatization Pa_{O_2} remains low, ventilation remains high, and therefore Pa_{CO_2} remains low. The kidneys act to lower plasma bicarbonate and return arterial pH toward normal. The oxygen content of arterial blood increases owing to an increase in hematocrit stimulated by the increased production of erythropoietin in the kidney.

237. The answer is D. *(Berne, 2/e. pp 620–622.)* End-pulmonary capillary blood normally reaches equilibrium with alveolar tensions of carbon dioxide, nitrogen, and oxygen. This is because the blood normally spends enough time in the pulmonary capillaries for these gases to reach equilibrium. If nitrous oxide (N_2O) is added to the inspired gas, it would also quickly reach equilibrium with pulmonary capillary blood. Oxygen takes longer than CO_2, N_2, or N_2O to reach equilibrium because a large amount of O_2 must diffuse into the blood to saturate the hemoglobin. In contrast, carbon monoxide, which is used at very low partial pressures to measure the diffusing capacity of the lung, does not have time to reach equilibrium in the time the blood spends in the pulmonary capillaries. This is because carbon monoxide so avidly binds to hemoglobin. The P_{CO} in the pulmonary capillary rises very slowly.

238. The answer is E. *(Berne, 2/e. pp 627–628, 636–639.)* In the graph accompanying the question, curve B shows a depressed ventilatory response to elevation of P_{CO_2}. The response would be produced by central nervous system depressants such as barbiturates, benzodiazepines such as diazepam (Valium), and narcotics such as morphine, as well as by diminished alertness (sleep), which would reflect the overall level of activity in the reticular activating system of the brainstem. The sensitivity of the respiratory center to P_{CO_2} may be increased during exercise.

239. The answer is B. *(West, 12/e. pp 562–566.)* Pulmonary compliance, defined as the ratio of change of lung volume to the change in pressure required to inflate the lung ($\Delta V/\Delta P$), is an index of lung distensibility. It decreases in patients with pulmonary edema and interstitial fibrosis and increases in patients with emphysema and in persons of advancing years. The stiffer the lung, the lower the pulmonary compliance. Surfactant lowers the surface tension in the alveoli and makes the lung more distensible.

240. The answer is A. *(Berne, 2/e. pp 627–630.)* The central chemoreceptors are located at or near the ventral surface of the medulla. They are stimulated to increase ventilation by a decrease in the pH of their extracellular fluid (ECF). The pH of this ECF is affected by the P_{CO_2} of the blood supply to the medullary chemoreceptor area as well as by the CO_2 and lactic acid production of the surrounding brain tissue. The central chemoreceptors are not stimulated by decreases in Pa_{O_2} or blood oxygen content but rather can be depressed by long-term or severe decreases in oxygen supply.

241. The answer is B. *(West, 12/e. pp 581–582, 584–585.)* Hypoxemia or a decreased arterial P_{O_2} stimulates the peripheral chemoreceptors in both the carotid and aortic bodies. Hypoxemia does not stimulate the central chemoreceptors. When Pa_{O_2} falls below about 60 mmHg, the chemoreceptor reflex mediated by the peripheral chemoreceptors in the carotid bodies causes ventilation to increase. The peripheral chemoreceptors also have an input into the vasomotor centers in the medulla. The net effect of hypoxemic stimulation of the peripheral chemoreceptors on the cardiovascular system is to cause a reflex increase in arterial blood pressure.

242. The answer is A. *(Berne, 2/e. pp 639–640. West, 12/e. pp 538–540, 588–592.)* At a high altitude, arterial P_{O_2} is low because of the low barometric pressure. Ventilation increases owing to stimulation of the carotid body chemoreceptors, and Pa_{O_2} increases somewhat, although it does not return to a normal, sea-level value. With this hyperventilation, Pa_{CO_2} decreases, resulting in a respiratory alkalosis that may become fully compensated with time via renal mechanisms. A lower-than-normal Pa_{CO_2} would shift the oxyhemoglobin dissociation curve to the left, thereby increasing the affinity of hemoglobin for oxygen. Chronic hypoxia at high altitudes or in disease states stimulates the increased release of erythropoietin from the kidneys, which increases the hematocrit and thereby increases the hemoglobin concentration of the blood. Thus at the same lowered Pa_{O_2}, the oxygen content of blood and oxygen delivery to tissues increase. Chronic hypoxia also stimulates increased capillary growth in tissues.

243. The answer is D. *(Berne, 2/e. pp 586–587. West, 12/e. pp 568–572.)* The tone of bronchial smooth muscle is under autonomic control. Stimulation of sympathetic nerves causes bronchodilation, whereas parasympathetic stimulation via the vagus nerve causes bronchoconstriction. Bronchoconstriction reduces the radius of the airways and thereby decreases anatomic dead space and increases airway resistance, which consequently increases the resistive work of breathing. Bronchoconstriction has no significant effect on the elastic properties of the lung.

244. The answer is D. *(Berne, 2/e. pp 629–631. West, 12/e. pp 581–583.)* Stimulation of the peripheral chemoreceptors, particularly the carotid bodies, causes an increase in ventilation that results in a decrease in Pa_{CO_2} (termed *hyperventilation*). Stimulation of other receptors in the body both within the lungs and elsewhere can affect ventilation and can override the normal chemical control of ventilation, thus causing either hyper- or hypoventilation. Stimulation of peripheral pain receptors tends to cause hyperventilation, whereas stimulation of visceral pain receptors tends to cause hypoventilation. Stimulation of irritant receptors (also called *rapidly adapting receptors*) and J (juxtacapillary) receptors generally causes rapid, shallow breathing, which can result in hyperventilation. Intense stimulation of J receptors can cause apnea. However, stimulation of the pulmonary stretch receptors terminates inspiration and alone would not be expected to cause hyperventilation.

245. The answer is B. *(West, 12/e. pp 533–534, 554–557, 574–575.)* There is a negative, or subatmospheric, intrapleural pressure (P_{IP}) between the lungs and the chest wall due to the tendency of the chest wall to pull outward and the tendency of the lungs to collapse. Because the lungs are essentially "hanging" in the chest, the force of gravity on the lungs causes the P_{IP} to be more negative at the top of the lung. This also causes the alveoli at the apex (top) of the lung to be larger than those at the base (bottom) of the lung. Larger alveoli are already more inflated and are less compliant than smaller alveoli. During inspiration, when all alveoli are subjected to essentially the same alveolar pressure, more air will go to the more compliant alveoli. Because of the effect of gravity on blood, more blood flow will go to the base of the lung. This does not appreciably affect lung compliance. Ventilation is about three times greater at the base of the lung, but flow is about ten times greater at the base than at the apex of the lung. Therefore, the V/Q ratio is lower at the base than at the apex in a normal lung.

246. The answer is D. *(West, 12/e. pp 242–243.)* A Swan-Ganz catheter can be floated in the pulmonary artery to measure pulmonary artery systolic and diastolic pressures and, if advanced far enough, pulmonary capillary wedge pressure. Pulmonary capillary wedge pressure is substantially lower than the mean pressure in the pulmonary artery and is an indirect measure of pulmonary venous and left atrial pressures. The Swan-Ganz catheter would not sense the aortic pressure, which is an order of magnitude higher than the pulmonary artery pressure.

247. The answer is B. *(West, 12/e. pp 522–524.)* A spirometer is an instrument that records the volume of air moved into and out of the lungs during respiration and thus would measure all lung volumes included in maximal inspiration or expiration. Residual volume, which is the volume of gas in the lungs after maximal expiration; functional residual capacity, which is residual volume plus expiratory reserve volume; and total lung capacity, which is the total volume of gas in the lungs after maximal inspiration, cannot be measured directly by a spirometer. They can be measured using a spirometer by gas dilution techniques or by body plethysmography.

248–255. The answers are: 248-B, 249-B, 250-E, 251-B, 252-C, 253-D, 254-D, 255-A. *(Ganong, 15/e. pp 627–628, 680–686. West, 12/e. pp 498–502.)* An increase in pH accompanied by a decrease in P_{CO_2} represents respiratory alkalosis, a situation that commonly accompanies hyperventilation. An increased respiratory rate at constant tidal volume or an increased tidal volume at constant respiratory rate would each increase alveolar ventilation. The actual increases in alveolar ventilation in those situations would differ slightly, owing to differences in volume of dead space ventilation. Hyperventilation can decrease arterial P_{CO_2} from 40 to 15 mmHg and elevate arterial P_{O_2} from 90 to 140 mmHg. After normal breathing is resumed, a period of apnea occurs followed by several short breaths and then another period of apnea, in cycles, until the normal pattern returns. This reflects the time required for reequilibration of arterial P_{CO_2} and the return of CO_2 regulation of the respiratory center. Respiratory alkalosis also occurs in persons living at high altitude. At high altitudes, low atmospheric P_{O_2} associated with diminished barometric pressure causes hypoxia-induced hyperventilation with eventual equilibration and return of pH to normal. The P_{CO_2} remains decreased, however, resulting in respiratory alkalosis.

Metabolic acidosis is a consequence of the addition to the blood of stronger acids than the body's natural buffer systems can neutralize. The accumulation of ketone bodies associated with diabetes mellitus is an example of metabolic acidosis; excess H^+ is buffered and the resulting H_2CO_3 is rapidly separated into CO_2 and water. The low blood pH stimulates the carotid bodies to produce hyperventilation and a reduction in P_{CO_2}.

Respiratory arrest, by definition, is associated with decreased ventilation. Extracellular fluid levels of CO_2 rise, increasing arterial P_{CO_2}. The CO_2 is converted to $H^+ + HCO_3^-$ and results in a decrease in pH, producing *respiratory* acidosis.

Administration of CO_2 will increase P_{CO_2} and lead to formation of H^+ from H_2CO_3 with a resultant decrease in pH. The increase in P_{CO_2} stimulates the respiratory center to increase ventilation.

An increase in pH with an increase in P_{CO_2} constitutes metabolic alkalosis. Metabolic alkalosis involves a reduction in free $[H^+]$ as a consequence of addition of alkali or removal of acid. The pH necessarily rises and acid-base balance is restored by compensatory hypoventilation, which produces an increase in P_{CO_2}. However, compensatory hypoventilation to the point of hypoxia does not occur.

In each of these situations involving changes in acid-base balance, renal mechanisms also play a role in reestablishing normal balance. Thus, in acidosis, there is an increase in H^+ excreted as $H_2PO_4^-$ and NH_4^+. In alkalosis, HCO_3^- excretion is favored.

256–264. The answers are: 256-C, 257-B, 258-A, 259-A, 260-E, 261-A, 262-A, 263-C, 264-D. *(Berne, 2/e. pp 609–612.)* The hemoglobin molecule consists of four globin chains, each of which contains one heme unit. Each heme contains one iron atom in the ferrous (Fe^{2+}) state and each can bind one O_2 molecule. The binding of an O_2 molecule to one heme facilitates the binding of O_2 to the others. This cooperative interaction results in the sigmoid shape of the normal oxyhemoglobin dissociation curve. As the Pa_{O_2} increases, the amount of O_2 bound to hemoglobin increases until the hemoglobin is saturated. The P_{O_2} at which the hemoglobin is 50 percent saturated with oxygen is called the P_{50}. In normal adult blood at pH 7.4 and 37°C, it is about 29 mmHg (curve B). The P_{50} is used as a measure of the affinity of hemoglobin for oxygen. Under different conditions, the oxyhemoglobin dissociation curve can be shifted to the left or right of normal (curve B); that is, the affinity of hemoglobin for O_2 can be increased or decreased. The curve is shifted to the right (curve C) when P_{CO_2} is increased, when pH is decreased, and when the temperature is increased. The curve is shifted to the left (curve A) by the conditions opposite to those that shift the curve to the right. Many shifts in the curve are phys-iologically advantageous. For example, in the peripheral tissues, oxygenated blood enters the tissue capillaries where the P_{CO_2} is higher and the pH is lower. These factors decrease the affinity of hemoglobin for oxygen and facilitate the unloading of O_2 from hemoglobin. In exercising muscle, in addition to these factors, there is also an increase in temperature that further facilitates O_2 unloading.

Within the red blood cells, there is a high concentration of 2,3-diphos-phoglycerate (2,3-DPG), which is formed from 1,3-DPG, a product of glycol-ysis. An increase in the amount of 2,3-DPG in the red cells causes the oxy-hemoglobin dissociation curve to shift to the right. A decrease in 2,3-DPG shifts the curve to the left. During chronic hypoxia, the amount of 2,3-DPG in the red cells increases. This facilitates O_2 unloading but can also hinder O_2 loading in the lungs if the hypoxia is severe enough. When blood is stored, the amount of 2,3-DPG falls, which shifts the curve to the left and hinders unloading of O_2.

In anemia (curve E), the hematocrit is reduced, thereby reducing the hemoglobin concentration and the oxygen capacity of the blood. The P_{50} is not different from that of normal blood but the oxygen content of the blood at any given P_{O_2} is less because of the decreased amount of hemoglobin.

Carbon monoxide (CO) binds to hemoglobin (HbCO) more than 200 times as avidly as oxygen. When CO binds to hemoglobin, it shifts the oxyhemo-globin dissociation curve to the left and makes it less sigmoid in shape (curve D). The presence of HbCO reduces the amount of hemoglobin available to bind to oxygen and the shift of the curve to the left hinders the unloading of the O_2 that does bind.

The globin chains of adult hemoglobin consist of two α and two β chains. Fetal hemoglobin has two α and two γ chains. Because of this difference, fetal hemoglobin does not bind 2,3-DPG and the fetal oxyhemoglobin dissociation curve is therefore shifted to the left (curve A) compared with the adult curve. The higher affinity for O_2 of the fetal hemoglobin facilitates the extraction of O_2 by the fetus from the maternal blood.

265–267. The answers are: 265-A, 266-B, 267-A. *(Berne, 2/e. pp 615–619. West, 12/e. pp 554–558.)* The ventilation-perfusion (V/Q) ratio is the ratio of the rate of alveolar ventilation to the rate of pulmonary blood flow. It is higher at the top of the lung than at the bottom of the lung. This is because ventilation is about 3 times higher at the bottom of the lung than at the top but perfusion is about 10 times higher at the bottom of the lung than at the top. Low V/Q areas result in blood with a lower-than-normal P_{O_2} and a higher-than-normal P_{CO_2}. High V/Q areas result in blood with a higher-than-normal P_{O_2} and a lower-than-normal P_{CO_2}. The mixing of blood from areas throughout the lung with different V/Q ratios is responsible for the alveolar-arterial oxygen (A-a) difference.

In a patient with a blocked right main bronchus, blood flowing through the right lung would not be oxygenated and would mix in the pulmonary veins with oxygenated blood coming from the left lung. Thus the Pa_{O_2} of the arterial blood would be lower than normal. Initially the Pa_{CO_2} would be increased, but the central and peripheral chemoreceptors would increase ventilation to bring Pa_{CO_2} back to normal. Pa_{O_2} would increase slightly but remain low because of the nonlinearity of the oxyhemoglobin dissociation curve.

268–269. The answers are: 268-C, 269-B. *(Berne, 2/e. pp 609–612. West, 12/e. pp 538–542.)* The *oxygen content* is defined as the total amount of oxygen contained in a given volume of blood. This includes dissolved oxygen, which constitutes a very small portion of the total oxygen, and oxygen bound to hemoglobin, which constitutes the bulk of the oxygen carried by blood. The partial pressure of oxygen determines both the amount of dissolved oxygen as well as the degree of oxygen saturation of hemoglobin. Thus, the oxygen content of blood depends on both the P_{O_2} and the concentration or amount of hemoglobin available to carry oxygen. The percentage of hemoglobin saturated by oxygen, however, is dependent only on the P_{O_2} and not on how much hemoglobin is present. Other factors such as pH, P_{CO_2}, and temperature affect the affinity of hemoglobin for oxygen and can therefore affect the percentage of saturation.

270–278. The answers are: 270-B, 271-A, 272-A, 273-A, 274-A, 275-B, 276-A, 277-C, 278-B. *(Ganong, 15/e. pp 604–608. West, 12/e. pp 562–566, 576–578.)* Restrictive pulmonary disease is manifested by a decrease in lung compliance; that is, there is a decreased change of lung volume per unit of change of pressure. There is an increase in the elastic recoil of the lungs, which makes them more difficult to expand. In the respiratory distress syndrome in the infant, a restrictive disease, there is an insufficient amount of surfactant in the alveoli. Surfactant is a phospholipid produced by type II granular pneumocytes in the walls of the alveoli. Surfactant reduces the surface tension of the fluid lining the alveoli. With too little surfactant present, the surface tension is high and tends to collapse the alveoli; this makes it harder to expand the lungs. Another example of a restrictive disease is lung fibrosis. In fibrosis the interstitial tissue of the lung itself becomes stiffer and harder to expand, which decreases lung compliance. Because of the increased elastic recoil of the lungs in restrictive disease, lung volumes are typically decreased. These include total lung capacity (TLC), vital capacity (VC), functional residual capacity (FRC), and residual volume (RV). Because the vital capacity is reduced, the FEV_1 (forced expiratory volume expelled in 1 s) is reduced. However, because of the increased lung recoil, the ratio FEV_1/VC is normal or greater than normal.

Examples of obstructive lung disease are asthma, bronchitis, and emphysema. In asthma there is a narrowing of the airways due to an increase in bronchial smooth muscle tone. In obstructive disease there is early closure of the airways during expiration, which traps gas in the lungs. In asthma and bronchitis this closure is due to narrowed airways and in emphysema it is due to a loss of elastic fibers in the lung. In patients with active obstructive disease, FRC and RV are increased. This is because of gas trapping in the lungs. In patients with emphysema, TLC is usually increased as well. Vital capacity is usually somewhat decreased. The FEV_1 is greatly decreased because of the decrease in vital capacity and because of increased early airway closure and gas trapping during a forced expiration. The ratio FEV_1/VC is well below normal.

The work of breathing is increased in disease but the breathing patterns minimize the increase in work. The work of breathing has two components: elastic work and resistive work. In restrictive disease where there are increased elastic forces to overcome, breathing is usually rapid and shallow, which minimizes the elastic work. In obstructive disease, breathing is usually slow and deep, which minimizes the resistive work of breathing.

Renal and Acid-Base Physiology

DIRECTIONS: Each question below contains five suggested responses. Select the **one best** response to each question.

279. The consumption of oxygen by the kidney

(A) decreases as blood flow increases
(B) is regulated by erythropoietin
(C) remains constant as blood flow increases
(D) directly reflects the level of sodium transport
(E) is greatest in the medulla

280. If the plasma concentration of a freely filterable substance that is neither secreted nor reabsorbed is 0.125 mg/mL, its urine concentration 25 mg/mL, and urine formation 1.0 mL/min, the glomerular filtration rate is

(A) 50 mL/min
(B) 125 mL/min
(C) 150 mL/min
(D) 200 mL/min
(E) 362 mL/min

281. Major determinants of plasma osmolarity include all the following EXCEPT

(A) sodium
(B) hemoglobin
(C) chloride
(D) albumin
(E) glucose

282. Metabolic alkalosis can be caused by all the following EXCEPT

(A) hyperaldosteronism
(B) hyperventilation
(C) hypokalemia
(D) volume depletion
(E) vomiting

283. An increase in the concentration of plasma potassium causes an increase in

(A) release of renin
(B) secretion of aldosterone
(C) secretion of ADH
(D) release of natriuretic hormone
(E) production of angiotensin II

284. The figures shown below depict the relationship of a substance's excretion rate (UV) and plasma clearance ($\frac{UV}{P}$) to its plasma concentration (U = urinary concentration, V = urinary flow rate, and P = plasma concentration). Based on these data, it can be seen that the substance is

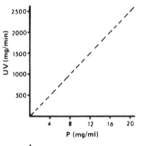

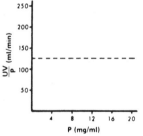

(A) not excreted in urine in proportion to its plasma concentration
(B) excreted in urine at a rate inversely proportional to its plasma concentration
(C) excreted in urine at a rate independent of its plasma concentration
(D) cleared from the body at a rate that decreases as its plasma concentration increases
(E) cleared from the body independently of its plasma concentration

285. In the graph below showing the tubular loss of glucose versus the tubular load of glucose, the transport maximum (Tm) for glucose is located at which of the following points?

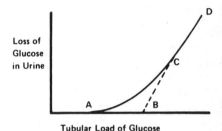

(A) A
(B) B
(C) C
(D) D
(E) None of the above

286. The syndrome of inappropriate antidiuretic hormone secretion (SIADH) is caused by the excess release of ADH. SIADH will have the LEAST effect on

(A) concentration of plasma sodium
(B) total body water
(C) urinary flow
(D) urinary osmolarity
(E) plasma osmolarity

287. Amino acids are almost completely reabsorbed from the glomerular filtrate via active transport in the

(A) proximal tubule
(B) loop of Henle
(C) distal tubule
(D) collecting duct
(E) renal pelvis

Questions 288–291

Use the Henderson equation or the Henderson-Hasselbalch equation to calculate the missing acid-base parameters.

288. Patient X was admitted to the hospital with a Pa_{CO_2} of 30 mmHg and an arterial $[H^+]$ of 50 nmol/L (pH 7.30). His plasma bicarbonate concentration is

(A) 7.2 mmol/L
(B) 14.4 mmol/L
(C) 30.0 mmol/L
(D) 40.0 mmol/L
(E) 62.5 mmol/L

289. Patient X from the previous question most likely has which of the following acid-base disorders?

(A) Metabolic acidosis
(B) Metabolic alkalosis
(C) Respiratory acidosis
(D) Respiratory alkalosis
(E) Mixed metabolic acidosis and respiratory acidosis

290. Patient Y has a Pa_{CO_2} of 30 mmHg and a plasma bicarbonate concentration of 22 mmol/L. What is her concentration of plasma hydrogen ion (pH)?

(A) 18 nmol/L; pH = 7.75
(B) 28 nmol/L; pH = 7.56
(C) 33 nmol/L; pH = 7.49
(D) 40 nmol/L; pH = 7.40
(E) 48 nmol/L; pH = 7.32

291. Patient Y from the previous question most likely has which of the following acid-base disorders?

(A) Metabolic acidosis
(B) Metabolic alkalosis
(C) Respiratory acidosis
(D) Respiratory alkalosis
(E) Mixed metabolic alkalosis and respiratory acidosis

292. The daily production of hydrogen ion from CO_2 is primarily buffered by

(A) extracellular bicarbonate
(B) red blood cell bicarbonate
(C) red blood cell hemoglobin
(D) plasma proteins
(E) plasma phosphate

293. Glomerular filtration rate would be increased by

(A) constriction of the afferent arteriole
(B) a decrease in afferent arteriolar pressure
(C) compression of the renal capsule
(D) a decrease in the concentration of plasma protein
(E) a decrease in renal blood flow

294. The following clinical laboratory data were obtained from a patient with diabetes mellitus: plasma $[Na^+]$ = 140 meq/L; plasma $[K^+]$ = 7.0 meq/L; plasma $[Cl^-]$ = 105 meq/L; plasma $[HCO_3^-]$ = 6 meq/L; arterial $[H^+]$ = 80 neq/L; plasma [glucose] = 600 mg/dL. Calculate the anion gap.

(A) 12 meq/L
(B) 22 meq/L
(C) 29 meq/L
(D) 36 meq/L
(E) 42 meq/L

295. The greatest amount of hydrogen ion secreted by the proximal tubule is associated with

(A) excretion of potassium ion
(B) excretion of hydrogen ion
(C) reabsorption of calcium ion
(D) reabsorption of bicarbonate ion
(E) reabsorption of phosphate ion

Questions 296–297

The following measurements are obtained from a patient: PAH clearance = 750 mL/min; plasma creatinine concentration = 0.8 mg/dL; urinary creatinine concentration = 66 mg/dL; urinary excretion = 2 mL/min; plasma glucose concentration = 120 mg/dL.

296. What is the patient's filtration fraction?

(A) 0.18
(B) 0.20
(C) 0.22
(D) 0.24
(E) 0.26

297. Approximately how much glucose is reabsorbed by this patient's kidneys?

(A) 0 mg/min
(B) 120 mg/min
(C) 165 mg/min
(D) 200 mg/min
(E) 320 mg/min

Questions 298–300

The following measurements are taken from a patient:

Urinary volume = 1.5 L/day
Urinary [HCO_3^-] = 4 meq/L
Urinary titratable
   acids = 10 meq/L urine
Urinary [NH_4^+] = 20 meq/L

298. What is the daily net acid excretion for this patient?

(A) 51 meq/day
(B) 39 meq/day
(C) 34 meq/day
(D) 30 meq/day
(E) 26 meq/day

299. How much new bicarbonate is being formed per day in this patient?

(A) 51 meq/day
(B) 39 meq/day
(C) 34 meq/day
(D) 30 meq/day
(E) 26 meq/day

300. Assuming production of a normal fixed acid load, what is this patient's acid-base status?

(A) Normal
(B) Respiratory acidosis
(C) Metabolic acidosis
(D) Respiratory alkalosis
(E) None of the above

301. The major source of the *total* daily acid load produced by the body is

(A) anaerobic metabolism
(B) aerobic metabolism
(C) phospholipid catabolism
(D) protein catabolism
(E) triglyceride catabolism

302. The following data are obtained: renal artery para-amino-hippuric acid concentration (A_{PAH}) = 0.05 mg/mL; renal vein PAH concentration (V_{PAH}) = 0.005 mg/mL; urinary PAH concentration (U_{PAH}) = 20 mg/mL; urinary flow rate = 2 mL/min. Renal plasma flow is closest to

(A) 500 mL/min
(B) 600 mL/min
(C) 700 mL/min
(D) 800 mL/min
(E) 900 mL/min

303. If a substance appears in the renal artery but not in the renal vein,

(A) its clearance is equal to the glomerular filtration rate
(B) it must be secreted by the kidney
(C) its urinary concentration must be higher than its plasma concentration
(D) its clearance is equal to the renal plasma flow
(E) none of the above are true

304. A freely filterable substance that is neither reabsorbed nor secreted has a renal artery concentration of 12 mg/mL and a renal vein concentration of 9 mg/mL. Calculate the filtration fraction (GFR/RPF).

(A) 0.05
(B) 0.15
(C) 0.25
(D) 0.35
(E) 0.45

305. All the following comparisons between the distal nephron and the proximal tubule are correct EXCEPT

(A) the distal nephron is less permeable to hydrogen ion than is the proximal tubule
(B) the distal nephron is more responsive to aldosterone than is the proximal tubule
(C) the distal nephron has a more negative intraluminal potential than does the proximal tubule
(D) the distal nephron secretes more potassium than does the proximal tubule
(E) the distal nephron secretes more hydrogen ion than does the proximal tubule

306. Destruction of the supraoptic nuclei of the brain will produce which of the following changes in urinary volume and concentration? (Assume that fluid intake equals fluid loss.)

(A) Increased urinary volume and a very dilute urine
(B) Increased urinary volume and a concentrated urine
(C) Decreased urinary volume and a very dilute urine
(D) Decreased urinary volume and a concentrated urine
(E) None of the above

307. Which one of the following returns closest to normal during chronic respiratory acidosis?

(A) Alveolar ventilation
(B) Arterial P_{CO_2}
(C) Arterial P_{O_2}
(D) Plasma concentration of bicarbonate
(E) Arterial concentration of hydrogen ion

308. The hypothalamus will effect the release of ADH in response to all the following stimuli EXCEPT

(A) dehydration
(B) severe hemorrhage
(C) decreased blood osmolarity
(D) pain, anxiety, or surgical stress
(E) nicotine

309. The pH of the tubular fluid in the distal nephron can be lower than that in the proximal tubule because

(A) a greater sodium gradient can be established across the wall of the distal nephron than across the wall of the proximal tubule
(B) more buffer is present in the tubular fluid of the distal nephron than in the proximal tubule
(C) more hydrogen ion is secreted into the distal nephron than into the proximal tubule
(D) the brush border of the distal nephron contains more carbonic anhydrase than that of the proximal tubule
(E) the tight junctions of the distal nephron are less leaky to solute than those of the proximal tubule

310. Which of the following statements about renin is true?

(A) It is secreted by cells of the proximal tubule
(B) Its secretion leads to loss of sodium and water from plasma
(C) Its secretion is stimulated by increased mean renal arterial pressure
(D) It converts angiotensinogen to angiotensin I
(E) It converts angiotensin I to angiotensin II

311. H^+ secretion in the distal nephron is enhanced by all the following EXCEPT

(A) an increase in the level of plasma aldosterone
(B) an increase in the tubular luminal concentration of poorly reabsorbable anions
(C) hyperkalemia
(D) metabolic acidosis
(E) respiratory acidosis

312. In controlling the synthesis and secretion of aldosterone, which of the following factors is LEAST important?

(A) Renin
(B) Angiotensin II
(C) Concentration of plasma Na^+
(D) Concentration of plasma K^+
(E) Adrenocorticotropic hormone (ACTH)

313. A patient is found to have a urine creatinine concentration of 196 mg/mL; a plasma creatinine concentration of 1.4 mg/mL; and a urine flow of 1 mL/min. The creatinine clearance is

(A) 75 mL/min
(B) 98 mL/min
(C) 125 mL/min
(D) 140 mL/min
(E) 196 mL/min

314. Renal correction of hyperkalemia will result in

(A) alkalosis
(B) acidosis
(C) increased secretion of HCO_3^-
(D) increased secretion of H^+
(E) increased excretion of Na^+

315. In 1 h, 54 mL of urine is collected from a test subject. The concentration of para-aminohippuric acid (PAH) in the plasma is 0.02 mg/mL, and in the urine it is 14 mg/mL. What is the effective renal plasma flow (ERPF)?

(A) 31.1 mL/min
(B) 128 mL/min
(C) 278 mL/min
(D) 630 mL/min
(E) 771 mL/min

316. Most of the glucose that is filtered through the glomerulus undergoes reabsorption in the

(A) proximal tubule
(B) descending limb of the loop of Henle
(C) ascending limb of the loop of Henle
(D) distal tubule
(E) collecting duct

317. When the potassium content of a patient's diet is increased fivefold, that patient is noted to have a change in concentration of plasma K^+ from 3.5 meq/L to 5 meq/L. The most likely explanation for this change is that

(A) the concentration of plasma K^+ is sensitive to dietary intake
(B) secretion of antidiuretic hormone is reduced
(C) the patient has an aldosterone-secreting tumor
(D) the patient has adrenal insufficiency
(E) the patient has renal insufficiency

318. Urinary volume is increased by all the following EXCEPT

(A) diabetes insipidus
(B) diabetes mellitus
(C) sympathetic stimulation
(D) increased renal arterial pressure
(E) infusion of mannitol

319. Which of the following structural features distinguishes the epithelial cells of the proximal tubule from those of the distal tubule?

(A) The distal tubule has a thicker basement membrane
(B) The proximal tubule has a thicker basement membrane
(C) The proximal tubule has a more extensive brush border
(D) The proximal tubule forms the juxtaglomerular apparatus
(E) The distal tubule has fewer tight intercellular junctions

320. Which of the following statements concerning the renal handling of proteins is correct?

(A) Proteins are more likely to be filtered if they are negatively charged than if they are uncharged
(B) Proteins can be filtered and secreted but not reabsorbed by the kidney
(C) Most of the protein excreted each day is derived from tubular secretion
(D) Protein excretion is directly related to plasma protein concentration
(E) Protein excretion is increased by sympathetic stimulation of the kidney

321. Glomerular filtration rate (GFR) and renal blood flow (RBF) will both be increased if

(A) the efferent and afferent arterioles are both dilated
(B) the efferent and afferent arterioles are both constricted
(C) only the afferent arteriole is constricted
(D) only the efferent arteriole is constricted
(E) the afferent arteriole is constricted and the efferent arteriole is dilated

322. Significant buffers for hydrogen ions generated in the body from anaerobic metabolism include all the following EXCEPT

(A) extracellular bicarbonate
(B) plasma proteins
(C) plasma lactate
(D) inorganic phosphates
(E) intracellular proteins

323. Extracellular bicarbonate ions serve as an effective buffer for all the following EXCEPT

(A) sulfuric acid
(B) phosphoric acid
(C) lactic acid
(D) carbonic acid
(E) β-hydroxybutyric acid

324. All the following statements are true of the H^+ secreted into the lumen of the distal nephron EXCEPT that it

(A) can combine with NH_4^+
(B) can combine with HCO_3^-
(C) can combine with HPO_4^{2-}
(D) can remain as free H^+
(E) is secreted by an H^+-ATPase pump

325. During chronic metabolic acidosis, all the following will occur EXCEPT

(A) all the filtered HCO_3^- will be reabsorbed by the kidney
(B) the production of ammonia by the kidney will increase
(C) H^+ secretion in the distal nephron will be enhanced
(D) glutamine uptake by the kidney will be enhanced
(E) the urinary pH will be increased

326. Aldosterone causes a decrease in the renal tubular secretion of

(A) magnesium
(B) hydrogen
(C) sodium
(D) potassium
(E) ammonium

327. A man drinks 2 L of water to replenish the fluids lost by sweating during a period of exercise. Compared with the situation prior to the period of sweating,

(A) his intracellular fluid will be hypertonic
(B) his extracellular fluid will be hypertonic
(C) his intracellular fluid volume will be greater
(D) his extracellular fluid volume will be greater
(E) his intracellular and extracellular fluid volumes will be unchanged

328. Ammonia is an effective and important urinary buffer for which of the following reasons?

(A) Its production in the kidney decreases during chronic acidosis
(B) The walls of the renal tubules are impermeable to NH_3
(C) The walls of the renal tubules are impermeable to NH_4^+
(D) Its acid-base reaction has a low pK_a
(E) None of the above

329. The amount of potassium excreted by the kidney will decrease if

(A) distal tubular flow increases
(B) circulating aldosterone levels increase
(C) dietary intake of potassium increases
(D) Na^+ reabsorption by the distal nephron decreases
(E) the excretion of organic ions increases

330. A respiratory acidosis that results in an increase in the concentration of hydrogen ion in arterial blood from 40 neq/L (pH 7.4) to 50 neq/L (pH 7.3) would

(A) stimulate the peripheral chemoreceptors
(B) decrease the amount of ammonium excreted in the urine
(C) inhibit the central chemoreceptors
(D) increase the pH of the urine
(E) decrease the concentration of HCO_3^- in arterial blood

331. In the presence of ADH, the distal nephron is LEAST permeable to

(A) water
(B) ammonia
(C) urea
(D) sodium
(E) carbon dioxide

332. Which of the following substances will be more concentrated at the end of the proximal tubule than at the beginning of the proximal tubule?

(A) Glucose
(B) Creatinine
(C) Sodium
(D) Bicarbonate
(E) Phosphate

333. When a person is dehydrated, hypotonic fluid will be found in the

(A) glomerular filtrate
(B) proximal tubule
(C) loop of Henle
(D) distal convoluted tubule
(E) collecting duct

334. The electrically neutral active transport of sodium from the lumen of the kidney occurs in the

(A) proximal tubule
(B) descending limb of the loop of Henle
(C) ascending limb of the loop of Henle
(D) cortical collecting duct
(E) medullary collecting duct

335. In metabolic acidosis caused by diabetic ketoacidosis, which of the following would be greater than normal?

(A) Concentration of plasma HCO_3^-
(B) Anion gap
(C) Arterial P_{CO_2}
(D) Plasma pH
(E) None of the above

336. Decreasing the resistance of the afferent arteriole in the glomerulus of the kidney will decrease

(A) the renal plasma flow
(B) the filtration fraction
(C) the oncotic pressure of the peritubular capillary blood
(D) the glomerular filtration rate
(E) none of the above

337. If GFR increases, proximal tubular reabsorption of salt and water will increase by a process called *glomerulotubular balance*. Contributions to this process include

(A) an increase in peritubular capillary hydrostatic pressure
(B) a decrease in peritubular sodium concentration
(C) an increase in peritubular oncotic pressure
(D) an increase in proximal tubular flow
(E) an increase in peritubular capillary flow

338. The glomerular filtration barrier is composed of all the following EXCEPT

(A) fenestrated capillary endothelium
(B) macula densa
(C) basement membrane
(D) podocytes
(E) mesangial cells

339. Renin release from the juxtaglomerular apparatus is inhibited by

(A) beta-adrenergic agonists
(B) prostaglandins
(C) aldosterone
(D) stimulation of the macula densa
(E) increased pressure within the afferent arterioles

340. All the following will cause an increase in reabsorption of bicarbonate in the kidney EXCEPT

(A) hyperaldosteronism
(B) hypercapnia
(C) hyperkalemia
(D) metabolic acidosis
(E) volume depletion

341. Patients with renal insufficiency develop very high plasma concentrations of urea (uremia) because of an increase in

(A) synthesis of urea by the liver
(B) reabsorption of urea by the proximal tubules
(C) secretion of urea by the distal tubules
(D) the glomerular filtration rate
(E) the renal blood flow

342. Which one of the following statements about aldosterone is correct?

(A) It produces its effect by activating cAMP
(B) It produces its effect by increasing membrane permeability to potassium
(C) It causes an increased reabsorption of hydrogen ion
(D) It has its main effect on the proximal tubule
(E) It is secreted in response to an increase in blood pressure

343. The amount of H^+ excreted as titratable acid bound to phosphate would be increased by all the following EXCEPT

(A) an increase in the amount of phosphate filtered at the glomerulus
(B) an increase in the pH of the urine
(C) an increase in the dietary intake of phosphate
(D) an increase in the level of plasma parathyroid hormone (PTH)
(E) a decrease in the renal tubular maximum (Tm) for phosphate reabsorption

344. Carbonic anhydrase plays an important role in all the following EXCEPT

(A) the renal handling of HCO_3^- within the cells of the proximal tubule
(B) the renal handling of HCO_3^- within the lumen of the proximal tubule
(C) the renal handling of HCO_3^- within the cells of the tubules of the distal nephron
(D) the renal handling of HCO_3^- within the lumen of the tubules of the distal nephron
(E) the gastric secretion of HCl by the parietal cells

345. The effect of antidiuretic hormone (ADH) on the kidney is to

(A) increase the permeability of the distal nephron to water
(B) increase the glomerular filtration rate
(C) increase the excretion of Na^+
(D) increase the excretion of water
(E) increase the diameter of the renal artery

346. In the distal tubules, sodium reabsorption is increased directly by increased

(A) sympathetic nerve stimulation of the kidney
(B) atrial natriuretic hormone secretion
(C) antidiuretic hormone secretion
(D) aldosterone secretion
(E) angiotensin secretion

347. Over a period of several hours, all the following processes will contribute to the maintenance of a near normal pH when fixed acids are added to the blood EXCEPT

(A) renal production of bicarbonate
(B) renal excretion of H^+
(C) intracellular buffering
(D) extracellular buffering
(E) decreased ventilation

348. The ability of the kidney to excrete a concentrated urine will increase if

(A) the permeability of the proximal tubule to water decreases
(B) the rate of blood flow through the medulla decreases
(C) the rate of flow through the loop of Henle increases
(D) the activity of the Na-K pump in the loop of Henle decreases
(E) the permeability of the collecting duct to water decreases

349. The glomerular filtration rate will increase if

(A) circulating blood volume increases
(B) the afferent arteriolar resistance increases
(C) the efferent arteriolar resistance decreases
(D) the plasma protein concentration decreases
(E) urine flow through the urethra is blocked

350. All the following statements about the fluid flowing through the juxta-medullary nephrons in the presence of ADH are correct EXCEPT

(A) the fluid is isotonic to plasma when it enters the loop of Henle
(B) the fluid is hypertonic to plasma as it passes from the descending limb of the loop of Henle to the ascending limb
(C) the fluid is isotonic to plasma when it leaves the loop of Henle
(D) the fluid is isotonic to plasma when it enters the collecting duct
(E) the fluid is hypertonic when it is excreted by the nephron

DIRECTIONS: Each group of questions below consists of lettered choices followed by a set of numbered items. For each numbered item select the **one** lettered choice with which it is **most** closely associated. Each lettered choice may be used **once, more than once, or not at all.**

Questions 351–352

For each of the two conditions that follows, select the lettered point on the accompanying graph with which it is most likely to be associated.

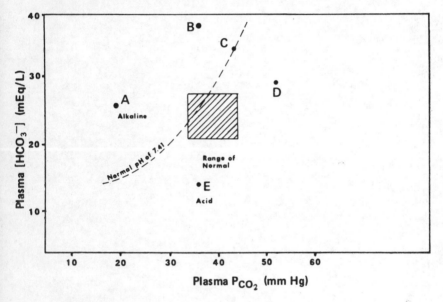

351. Uncompensated metabolic acidosis

352. Uncompensated respiratory alkalosis

Questions 353–357

For each of the following conditions, select the point on the accompanying graph with which it is most likely to be associated.

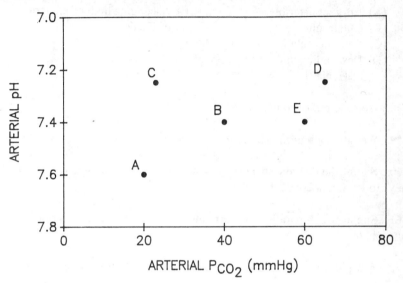

353. Metabolic acidosis

354. Acute respiratory acidosis

355. Acute respiratory alkalosis

356. Chronic respiratory acidosis

357. Ascent to high altitude

Questions 358–362

Match each of the descriptions below with the appropriate region of the kidney.

(A) Afferent arteriole
(B) Glomerulus
(C) Proximal tubule
(D) Descending limb of the loop of Henle

(E) Ascending limb of the loop of Henle
(F) Macula densa
(G) Vasa rectae
(H) Collecting duct

358. Isotonic reabsorption of sodium

359. Site at which permeability to water varies with plasma osmolarity

360. Site of the active transport system that makes it possible for the kidneys to excrete a concentrated urine

361. Site at which parathyroid hormone (PTH) regulates reabsorption of phosphate

362. A capillary network that is found only in the cortex of the kidney

Renal and Acid-Base Physiology

Answers

279. The answer is D. *(Ganong, 15/e. p 655. West, 12/e. p 436.)* In the kidney, oxygen is used primarily to support active transport of solutes, especially sodium, out of the tubules. In fact, oxygen consumption by the kidney is directly proportional to the amount of sodium reabsorbed and is greatest in the cortex where most tubular reabsorption of sodium occurs. An increase in renal blood flow will raise the glomerular filtration rate and increase the quantity of solute to be transported, so that oxygen consumption increases as blood flow increases and the arteriovenous oxygen difference remains constant. This is in contrast to the situation in other organs where increases in blood flow are accompanied by a decrease in arteriovenous oxygen difference. Erythropoietin is released in response to renal hypoxia and acts to increase erythrocyte production.

280. The answer is D. *(Ganong, 15/e. pp 655–656. Guyton, 8/e. pp 306–307.)* The glomerular filtration rate (GFR) is the volume of filtrate passing through all the nephrons each minute. It is influenced by the rate of blood flow through glomerular capillaries and by the permeability of the glomerular capillary wall and basement membrane. By using inulin, which is freely filtered and not reabsorbed or secreted, it is possible to determine the rate at which plasma passes through the glomerulus by comparing the rate of urinary excretion (urine volume × urinary concentration) with the plasma concentration, inasmuch as the filtered load equals the excreted load. Thus, for the example presented in the question,

$$\text{GFR} = \frac{25 \text{ mg/mL} \times 1 \text{ mL/min}}{0.125 \text{ mg/mL}} = 200 \text{ mL/min.}$$

281. The answer is B. *(West, 12/e. pp 412–418.)* The osmolarity of a solution or body fluid is determined by the number of osmotically active solute particles and not their size. In plasma and other extracellular fluid compartments, sodium and chloride ions are the major osmotically active substances. Glucose and albumin are present in much lower concentrations but make a sig-

133

nificant contribution to plasma osmolarity. Hemoglobin, being an intracellular protein, would not influence plasma osmolarity.

282. The answer is B. *(Rose, 3/e. pp 478–488.)* Metabolic alkalosis is caused by the loss of nonvolatile, or fixed, acid from the body. This can be by loss of H^+ from the gastrointestinal tract such as in vomiting of gastric acid. The loss of acid can also be from the kidneys. During volume depletion and hyperaldosteronism, plasma levels of aldosterone are elevated. Aldosterone, which increases renal sodium reabsorption, also increases renal H^+ secretion and excretion. During hypokalemia, K^+ moves out of cells in part in exchange for H^+ ions. This acidifies the renal tubular cells and increases renal H^+ secretion and excretion. Hyperventilation causes a respiratory alkalosis by decreasing arterial P_{CO_2} and results in the loss of volatile acid from the body.

283. The answer is B. *(Guyton, 8/e. pp 326–328.)* Aldosterone is the major hormone controlling the secretion of potassium by the distal tubule. It enhances the permeability of the luminal membrane to potassium, thus increasing the flow of potassium from the epithelial cells of the nephron, and increases the activity of the basolateral Na-K pump, thus increasing the movement of potassium from the interstitium to the epithelial cells. Potassium acts directly on the adrenal gland to increase the production and release of aldosterone.

284. The answer is E. *(Guyton, 8/e. pp 306–307.)* The top figure shown in the question demonstrates that the rate of excretion of a particular substance is directly proportional to, and a linear function of, its plasma concentration. The bottom figure shows that the substance's clearance $\frac{(UV)}{P}$ is constant and independent of the plasma concentration. These data are characteristic of inulin and indicate that the clearance of inulin equals the glomerular filtration rate.

285. The answer is B. *(Ganong, 15/e. pp 660–662. Guyton, 8/e. pp 305–306.)* Active tubular reabsorption of glucose is limited by a transport maximum (Tm), which depends on the level at which saturation of the transport mechanism occurs. When the filtered load exceeds the transport maximum, the excess is not reabsorbed but is excreted. Above the Tm, glucose excretion is directly related to filtered load (points C and D in the graph accompanying the question). In the curve exhibiting glucose tubular loss versus tubular load, the Tm is determined by extrapolation of the linear portion of the curve to the tubular load axis. The splay of the curve results from the fact that the tubules are not uniform and that at glucose levels *below* Tm, transport is partially reversible and therefore not all glucose is reabsorbed.

286. The answer is B. *(Guyton, 8/e. pp 314–315.)* Antidiuretic hormone (ADH) increases the permeability of the distal nephron to water. In high concentrations it also has a vasopressor effect (from which its other name, *arginine vasopressin,* is obtained). The increase in water permeability increases the amount of water reabsorbed from the distal nephron, thus producing a large decrease in urinary flow and a large increase in urinary osmolarity. The excess reabsorption of water produces a marked decrease in concentration of plasma sodium and osmolarity. Total body water increases very little because other regulatory mechanisms, for example the renin-angiotensin-aldosterone axis and atrial natriuretic hormone (ANH), keep body water close to normal.

287. The answer is A. *(Guyton, 8/e. pp 301–302.)* Amino acids are almost completely reabsorbed in the proximal renal tubules, along with glucose, proteins, acetoacetate ions, and vitamins. Very little of these substances is left in the tubular fluid entering the loop of Henle. Proteins, owing to their large size, are absorbed by pinocytosis through the proximal tubules' brush borders.

288–291. The answers are: 288-B, 289-A, 290-C, 291-D. *(Berne, 2/e. pp 806–813. Rose, 3/e. pp 270–272, 469–473.)* The Henderson and Henderson-Hasselbalch equations for the bicarbonate buffer system are used to evaluate acid-base status. The Henderson equation is

$$[H^+] \text{ (in nmol/L)} = 24 \times \frac{Pa_{CO_2} \text{ (in mmHg)}}{[HCO_3^-] \text{ (in mmol/L)}}$$

The conversion factors for the units and the K_a are "contained" in the number 24. The Henderson-Hasselbalch equation is the logarithmic form of this equation:

$$pH = 6.10 + \log \left(\frac{[HCO_3^-] \text{ (in mmol/L)}}{0.03 \dfrac{mmol/L}{mmHg} \times Pa_{CO_2} \text{ (in mmHg)}} \right)$$

The normal values are $[H^+]$ = 40 nmol/L, pH = 7.40, Pa_{CO_2} = 40 mmHg, and $[HCO_3^-]$ = 24 mmol/L. In practice it is easier to use the Henderson equation. For patient X the following would result:

$$50 \text{ nmol/L} = 24 \times \frac{30 \text{ mmHg}}{[HCO_3^-]}$$

$$[HCO_3^-] = 14.4 \text{ mmol/L}$$

Patient X has a higher-than-normal concentration of H^+ ion (a lower-than-normal pH). This indicates that an acidosis is present. He also has a lower-than-normal Pa_{CO_2}, which indicates he is hyperventilating. His bicarbonate level is also low. He most likely has a metabolic acidosis. Bicarbonate was consumed in the buffering of fixed acid. The Pa_{CO_2} is low because of stimulation of ventilation by the low arterial pH (respiratory compensation).

The following results can be obtained for patient Y:

$$[H^+] = 24 \times \frac{30 \text{ mmHg}}{22 \text{ mmol/L}}$$

$$[H^+] = 33 \text{ nmol/L (pH = 7.49)}$$

Patient Y has a lower-than-normal concentration of H^+ ion (higher-than-normal pH) and therefore has an alkalosis. Since the Pa_{CO_2} is lower than normal, the patient is hyperventilating and the alkalosis is therefore a respiratory alkalosis. The bicarbonate concentration is only slightly below normal and this reduction is due to the decrease in Pa_{CO_2} (acute respiratory alkalosis). Over time, if the hyperventilation continues, the kidneys would excrete bicarbonate and further reduce the plasma bicarbonate level to raise the arterial $[H^+]$ back toward normal (chronic respiratory alkalosis).

292. The answer is C. *(Ganong, 15/e. pp 619–621.)* Aerobic metabolism produces 13,000 to 24,000 mmol CO_2 per day. This yields close to that amount of H^+ ions produced per day via the reaction $CO_2 + H_2O \rightleftharpoons H_2CO_3 \rightleftharpoons H^+ + HCO_3^-$. At the tissues, CO_2 diffuses into the red cells, where the enzyme carbonic anhydrase accelerates the above reaction. The H^+ produced is buffered mainly by the large amount of hemoglobin in the red blood cells. Bicarbonate is not an effective buffer of volatile acid (from CO_2).

293. The answer is D. *(Berne, 2/e. pp 752–756.)* Glomerular filtration rate (GFR) will increase if there is an increase in the net glomerular capillary pres-

sure or the flow of fluid through the glomerulus. The net glome̸͟ͅr̸ capillary
pressure (or Starling forces) is equal to the glomerular capillar̸ ssure minus the sum of the plasma oncotic pressure and intrarenal pres̸ onstric-
tion of the afferent arteriole decreases glomerular capillary j̸ while
compression of the renal capsule increases the intrarenal pre̸ʲ oth of
these will cause a decrease in GFR. In contrast, decreasing the̸ ation
of plasma protein will decrease the plasma oncotic pressure ḙ o an
increase in GFR.

294. The answer is C. *(Rose, 3/e. pp 506–508.)* The anion gap
difference between the plasma concentration of sodium, the n̸e
the plasma, and the sum of the concentrations of plasma chlor̸
bonate, the major measured anions in the plasma.

$$\text{Anion gap} = [Na^+] - ([Cl^-] + [HCO_3^-])$$
$$= 140 \text{ meq/L} - (105 \text{ meq/L} + 6 \text{ meq/l})$$
$$= 29 \text{ meq/L}$$

The normal plasma concentrations of Na^+, Cl^-, and HCO_3^- are̸
105 meq/L, and 24 meq/L, respectively. The normal anion gap is f̸
meq/L. The anion gap is elevated when the concentration of unmea̸
ions in the plasma increases—for example, in cases of metabolic acid̸
as diabetic ketoacidosis and lactic acidosis. It is not elevated in m̸
acidosis caused by diarrhea.

295. The answer is D. *(Ganong, 15/e. pp 669–671.)* In the proximal tub̸
large amount of H^+ ion is secreted into the tubule lumen via an Na^+/
antiporter (exchanger). Most of this H^+ combines with bicarbonate ion in ̸
tubular fluid to form CO_2 and water. The CO_2 diffuses into the proximal t̸
bular cells, where the opposite reaction takes place to form H^+ and HCO_3^-
The HCO_3^- exits the cells on the basolateral side and enters the blood as
reabsorbed bicarbonate. Carbonic anhydrase is located on the luminal surface
of the cells as well as inside the cells to facilitate the above reactions.

296–297. The answers are: 296-C, 297-D. *(Guyton, 8/e. pp 304–307.)* The filtration fraction is the fraction of plasma filtered from the plasma flowing
through the kidney, or GFR/RPF. Renal plasma flow is equal to the clearance

R is equal to the clearance of creatinine. Clearance of creatinine
of PAH lated using the following formula:
can be

$$C_{cr} = \frac{U_{cr} \times \dot{V}}{P_{cr}}$$

$$= \frac{66 \times 2}{0.8}$$

$$= 165 \text{ mL/min}$$

filtration fraction = 165/750 = 0.22. At glucose concentrations be-
to 200 mg/dL, the kidneys will reabsorb all the glucose passing
the kidney. The filtered load of glucose = $P_{glu} \times$ GFR = 120 mg/dL
mL/min = 198 mg/min. Since all of this will be reabsorbed, the kidneys
rb approximately 200 mg of glucose per minute.

00. The answers are: 298-B, 299-B, 300-D. *(Ganong, 15/e. pp 669–671,*
682. Guyton, 8/e. pp 335–339.) Net acid excretion is equal to the sum of
amount of titratable acids plus the amount of the ammonium ions minus
amount of bicarbonate ions contained in the volume of urine produced
day.

$$\text{Net acid excretion} = ([\text{titratable acids}] + [NH_4^+] - [HCO_3^-]) \times \text{urine}$$
$$\text{volume per day}$$
$$= (10 \text{ meq/L} + 20 \text{ meq/L} - 4 \text{ meq/L}) \times 1.5 \text{ L/day}$$
$$= 39 \text{ meq/day}$$

Acid is excreted in urine bound to titratable acids, principally phosphates, and bound to ammonia as NH_4^+. If bicarbonate is present in urine,
its amount must be subtracted because a bicarbonate ion excreted in the urine
means that a hydrogen ion was left behind in the body. Conversely, a net
hydrogen ion excreted means that a bicarbonate ion was left behind in the
body. Thus, net acid excretion is equal to new bicarbonate formation.

The normal fixed acid production is 70 to 100 meq/day. This is eliminated
by the kidneys. This patient excreted only 39 meq H^+ per day and is therefore
conserving hydrogen ions. He is also excreting HCO_3^- (retaining H^+) and
must therefore be in a state of respiratory alkalosis. In respiratory and metabolic acidoses, the excretion of H^+ ion by the kidney is increased above normal and no bicarbonate ion is excreted in the urine.

301. The answer is B. *(Ganong, 15/e. pp 619–621. Guyton, 8/e. pp 334–335.)* Acid is produced in the body as volatile acid and nonvolatile, or fixed, acid. Volatile acid is from the CO_2 produced by aerobic metabolism in the mitochondria. This amounts to 13,000 to 24,000 mmol CO_2 and consequently H^+ per day. $CO_2 + H_2O \rightleftharpoons H_2CO_3 \rightleftharpoons H^+ + HCO_3^-$. In the lungs this CO_2 is blown off, thus eliminating the bulk of acid produced in the body. The fixed acids produced from other reactions in the body such as anaerobic metabolism and phospholipid and protein catabolism amount to 70 to 100 mmol per day and are excreted by the kidneys.

302. The answer is E. *(Berne, 2/e. pp 381–382. Rose, 3/e. pp 69–70.)* The clearance of PAH is a good estimate of renal plasma flow (RPF) because, under normal circumstances, almost all (more than 90 percent) the PAH passing through the kidney is excreted. However, less than 90 percent of the PAH might be reabsorbed in a diseased kidney. An accurate measure of RPF can be obtained from the formula

$$RPF = \frac{U_{PAH} \times \dot{V}}{A_{PAH} - V_{PAH}}$$

303. The answer is E. *(Rose, 3/e. pp 33–38, 69–70.)* If a substance disappears from the circulation during its passage through the kidney, it usually indicates that it has been secreted into the nephron. However, if the material is metabolized by the kidney, it may disappear without being secreted. If it is metabolized, then it will not appear in the urine and its clearance will have no relation to RPF. Even if it is entirely secreted by the kidney, its urinary concentration may be less than its plasma concentration if the urinary flow rate is very high.

304. The answer is C. *(Berne, 2/e. pp 780–784.)* Since the amount of fluid excreted by the kidney is only a small fraction of the renal plasma flow, the volume of fluid in the vein is essentially equal to that in the artery. Thus the difference in concentration must be due to the loss of solute. Since the material is neither reabsorbed nor secreted, its removal from the plasma must have been by glomerular filtration. Given that the filtered solute was 3 mg/mL and the renal artery concentration was 12 mg/mL, the fraction of solute filtered (and thus the fraction of solvent filtered) was 3/12 or 0.25.

305. The answer is E. *(Rose, 3/e. pp 139–141, 290–295, 303–304, 340.)* The distal nephron is less permeable to most solutes than is the proximal tubule because of the presence of large numbers of tight junctions connecting the epithelial cells to each other. Because of its low permeability the reabsorption of sodium, under the influence of aldosterone, generates a much more negative diffusion potential than can be produced in the proximal tubule. The proximal tubule reabsorbs about 60 percent of the filtered load of potassium. Almost all the remainder is reabsorbed in the loop of Henle. As a result, the amount of potassium excretion necessary to maintain potassium balance depends on the amount secreted in the distal nephron. Although more of the hydrogen secreted by the distal nephron is excreted, the proximal tubule secretes more. Almost all the hydrogen secreted by the proximal tubule is reclaimed in the reabsorption of bicarbonate.

306. The answer is A. *(Berne, 2/e. pp 924–928.)* Destruction of the supraoptic nuclei eliminates antidiuretic hormone (ADH) production. In the absence of ADH, the collecting ducts of the kidney would be impermeable to water and the final urine would be as dilute as the fluid leaving the ascending limb of the loop of Henle. In the absence of increased fluid intake, loss of water in excess of solute would result in increased osmolarity of body fluid. To maintain normal osmolarity, fluid intake must be increased. The increased fluid intake results in increased urinary volume because no water is conserved.

307. The answer is E. *(Berne, 2/e. p 813. Rose, 3/e. pp 560–565.)* Respiratory acidosis is caused by hypoventilation, i.e., a decrease in alveolar ventilation. When alveolar ventilation initially decreases (acute respiratory acidosis), arterial P_{CO_2} increases, arterial pH decreases (plasma [H^+] increases), and arterial P_{O_2} decreases. If the hypoventilation persists, the kidneys act to increase the concentration of plasma bicarbonate and excrete H^+ ions to bring the arterial concentration of hydrogen ion (pH) back toward or to normal. Alveolar ventilation, arterial P_{CO_2}, and arterial P_{O_2} remain abnormal.

308. The answer is C. *(Berne, 2/e. pp 924–928.)* Release of antidiuretic hormone (ADH) is controlled primarily by osmotic stimulation of the supraoptic nuclei of the hypothalamus. Because the effect of ADH is conservation of water for the maintenance of normal osmolarity, it follows that an increase and not a decrease in blood osmolarity would evoke ADH release. The other major stimulus to ADH secretion is reduction of effective plasma volume. Dehydration and hemorrhage both represent situations in which extracellular fluid volume would be decreased and conservation of water required. Pain and other neural stimuli, as well as pharmacologic agents such as nicotine and acetylcholine, also can promote ADH release.

309. The answer is E. *(Berne, 2/e. pp 798–799. Rose, 3/e. pp 290–295.)* The pH of the tubular fluid in the distal nephron can be lower than that in the proximal tubule because the tight junctions between the cells in the distal nephron are "tighter," or less leaky, than those in the proximal tubule. An H^+ ion gradient of only 10 to 1 (i.e., a minimum luminal pH of about 6.4) can be established in the proximal tubule, whereas an H^+ ion gradient of 1000 to 1 (i.e., a minimum luminal pH of 4.4) can be established in the distal nephron. Because of the tighter junctions, the distal nephron can also establish a greater sodium gradient. Even though the distal nephron can maintain a lower luminal pH, a lesser volume of H^+ ions is actually secreted than in the proximal tubule. The distal nephron, unlike the proximal tubule, does not have a true brush border and there is no carbonic anhydrase on the luminal surface of the cells as in the proximal tubule.

310. The answer is D. *(Berne, 2/e. pp 785–787, 969–970. Ganong, 15/e. pp 428–430.)* Renin is secreted by the juxtaglomerular cells (near the afferent arterioles) in response to decreased renal arterial pressure. It acts on angiotensinogen to form angiotensin I. Angiotensin I is then converted to angiotensin II, a highly potent pressor agent that, despite a short half-life in humans, has numerous regulator functions, including the control of aldosterone secretion and sodium and water conservation.

311. The answer is C. *(Rose, 3/e. pp 304–313.)* H^+ secretion in the distal nephron is enhanced by acidification of the cells of the tubules. This occurs during both metabolic and respiratory acidosis. It also occurs during hypokalemia as H^+ from outside the cells exchanges for K^+ from inside the cells. The opposite occurs in hyperkalemia. Thus, renal H^+ secretion is diminished in hyperkalemia. Aldosterone directly stimulates H^+ secretion by the distal nephron, and by strongly stimulating Na^+ reabsorption it also enhances the negative potential in the tubular lumen. Similarly, the presence of poorly reabsorbable anions in the lumen enhances the negative potential, and this negativity aids in the secretion of the H^+ cations into the lumen.

312. The answer is E. *(Berne, 2/e. pp 774–775, 969–973. West, 12/e. pp 481–483.)* The synthesis and secretion of aldosterone are dependent primarily upon the renin-angiotensin system. Decreased sodium concentration and increased potassium concentration stimulate aldosterone secretion in the absence of changes in plasma volume. The role of adrenocorticotropic hormone (ACTH) in aldosterone synthesis and secretion is negligible.

313. The answer is D. *(Ganong, 15/e. pp 655–656. Rose, 3/e. pp 64–68.)* The clearance of a substance by the kidney represents the volume of plasma from which the substance is completely removed, or cleared, per unit time. For creatinine,

$$\text{Creatinine clearance} = \frac{\text{Urine creatinine concentration} \times \text{urine flow}}{\text{Plasma creatinine concentration}}$$

$$= \frac{196 \text{ mg/mL} \times 1 \text{ mL/min}}{1.4 \text{ mg/mL}}$$

$$= 140 \text{ mL/min}.$$

Because creatinine tubular reabsorption and secretion are roughly equivalent, creatinine clearance may be regarded as a close approximation of glomerular filtration rate as measured more accurately with inulin.

314. The answer is B. *(Ganong, 15/e. pp 673–674.)* Hyperkalemia produces an increase in aldosterone secretion by the adrenal cortex. Aldosterone acts on the distal tubule to increase sodium reabsorption and decrease sodium excretion, as well as to enhance potassium secretion. When potassium excretion in the distal tubule is enhanced, hydrogen ion secretion, which also occurs in exchange for sodium resorption, is diminished. This reflects intracellular alkalosis, which occurs with hyperkalemia as cells lose hydrogen ion to take up potassium. As hydrogen ion secretion diminishes, hydrogen ion is retained and acidosis ensues.

315. The answer is D. *(Berne, 2/e. pp 780–784. Ganong, 15/e. pp 653–654.)* Effective renal plasma flow (ERPF) can be measured by determining the amount of an inert substance (not metabolized or stored in the kidney) excreted in the urine per unit time divided by the difference in its concentration in renal arterial blood and renal venous blood. Para-aminohippuric acid (PAH) is filtered readily and is also secreted by the renal tubule so that less than 10 percent of the filtered load is present in blood leaving the kidney. Thus, since its renal venous concentration would be negligible and its peripheral venous concentration would be identical to renal arterial concentration, the clearance of PAH would be a close approximation of ERPF. In the example given in the question,

$$\text{ERPF} = \frac{\text{Concentration of PAH in urine} \times \text{urine flow rate}}{\text{Concentration of PAH in plasma}}$$

$$= \frac{14 \text{ mg/mL} \times 54 \text{ mL/60 min}}{0.02 \text{ mg/mL}}$$

$$= 630 \text{ mL/min}.$$

Actual renal plasma flow would then be

$$\frac{ERPF}{PAH\ extraction} = \frac{630\ mL/min}{0.9} = 700\ mL/min$$

and

$$Renal\ blood\ flow = \frac{RPF}{1 - Hct} = \frac{700\ mL/min}{0.55} = 1270\ mL/min.$$

316. The answer is A. *(Berne, 2/e. pp 761–764. Ganong, 15/e. pp 660–662.)* Glucose reabsorption employs an active transport mechanism located in the proximal tubule. The same mechanism also transports fructose, galactose, and xylose. Essentially all filtered glucose is reabsorbed, inasmuch as the transport maximum (Tm) for glucose (320 mg/min) is not exceeded in normal persons. In diabetes mellitus, hyperglycemia results in a tubular filtration load that exceeds the Tm, and glycosuria ensues.

317. The answer is D. *(Guyton, 8/e. pp 326–328.)* Extracellular (plasma) K^+ concentration is maintained within a very narrow range despite wide fluctuations in dietary K^+ intake. This is a result of the fact that secretion of aldosterone by the adrenal cortex is very sensitive to small changes in K^+ concentration. Increased aldosterone secretion causes increased K^+ excretion by the distal tubule and would tend to reduce concentration of plasma K^+. In adrenal insufficiency, in which the regulatory function of aldosterone is absent, concentration of plasma K^+ can rise to very high levels and cause cardiac arrest. ADH secretion is not involved in the regulation of concentration of plasma K^+ but responds to changes in extracellular osmolality, which is determined largely by concentration of plasma Na^+.

318. The answer is C. *(Guyton, 8/e. pp 292–295, 308–309, 350–351.)* The rate of fluid volume excretion is influenced by the glomerular filtration rate (GFR) and the rate of tubular reabsorption. Increased renal arterial pressure increases urinary volume by increasing GFR, whereas sympathetic stimulation, by causing vasoconstriction, decreases both GFR and urinary volume. An increase in the filtered load of an osmotically active solute that is not reabsorbed, such as the nonmetabolized carbohydrate mannitol, or that is filtered in excess of the tubular capacity, such as glucose in diabetes mellitus, will decrease water resorption in parallel, and an osmotic diuresis will ensue. In diabetes insipidus, ADH secretion is markedly reduced or absent and water passes through the relatively impermeable collecting ducts without being reabsorbed.

319. The answer is C. *(Guyton, 8/e. pp 301–305.)* The major structural differences between epithelial cells of the proximal and distal tubules account for the fact that 65 percent of glomerular filtrate is reabsorbed in the proximal tubule and that the proximal tubule is more permeable to water. The proximal tubule has an extensive brush border composed of numerous microvilli, which markedly increase the surface area for reabsorption, and the tubule also has an extensive network of intracellular channels. The distal tubule has many more tight junctions between cells, which makes it less permeable to water. No significant difference in basement membrane thickness is observed between the proximal and distal tubules. The juxtaglomerular apparatus is formed by cells of the distal tubule lying adjacent to the afferent arteriole.

320. The answer is E. *(Berne, 2/e. pp 753–754. West, 12/e. pp 429–430, 456.)* Approximately two-thirds of the 40 to 150 mg of protein excreted per day by the kidney is derived from plasma proteins. The remainder is derived from the tubular secretion of a mucoprotein, the Tamm-Horsfall protein that is present in tubular casts appearing in urinary sediment. Not all plasma proteins are filtered equally because glomerular permeability is related to molecular size and charge. The larger and negatively charged proteins are poorly filtered. Most of the filtered protein is reabsorbed in the proximal tubule unless the filtered load exceeds the tubular capacity. Such overload would occur following damage to the glomerular basement membrane and breakdown of normal barriers, or following an increase in the plasma concentration of a small protein, such as myoglobin. Protein excretion is also increased by sympathetic stimulation, such as that occurring during exercise. In this situation, renal vasoconstriction reduces the glomerular filtration rate, which, by increasing the transit time of glomerular filtrate, favors diffusion of proteins across the basement membrane.

321. The answer is A. *(Berne, 2/e. pp 755–756. West, 12/e. pp 432–433.)* Renal blood flow is determined by the renal artery pressure and the resistance of the renal vascular bed. Decreasing the resistance of either the afferent or efferent arterioles could increase RBF. Alternatively, if the resistance of one of these vessels decreased more than the resistance of the other one increased, RBF would also increase. Glomerular filtration rate will increase if glomerular capillary pressure increases. This can occur if the afferent arteriolar resistance decreases or if the efferent arteriolar resistance increases.

322. The answer is C. *(Ganong, 15/e. pp 619–621, 682–683.)* Lactic acid, a fixed acid, is the product of anaerobic metabolism. Hydrogen ions from fixed acids produced in the body, such as lactic acid and ketone acids, are buffered by all available body buffers. They are buffered principally by bicarbonate through the reaction $H^+ + HCO_3^- \rightleftharpoons H_2CO_3 \rightleftharpoons CO_2 + H_2O$. The CO_2 produced is eliminated by the lungs. H^+ is later excreted by the kidney and HCO_3^- is added back to the plasma. Other body buffers are plasma proteins and intracellular proteins, including hemoglobin and inorganic phosphates. Lactate would not be a significant buffer as the acid produced is lactic acid.

323. The answer is D. *(Ganong, 15/e. pp 619–621, 681–683.)* The bicarbonate buffer system is of major importance in the buffering of fixed acids produced in the body, such as sulfuric acid, phosphoric acid, lactic acid, and ketone acids (e.g., β-hydroxybutyric acid). The reaction is $H^+ + HCO_3^- \rightleftharpoons H_2CO_3 \rightleftharpoons CO_2 + H_2O$. Bicarbonate is ineffective in buffering acid produced from CO_2, e.g., carbonic acid (H_2CO_3), because CO_2 is a product of the buffering reaction.

324. The answer is A. *(Ganong, 15/e. pp 619–621, 669–671.)* H^+ is secreted into the lumen of the distal tubule by an electrogenic H^+ ion pump. This H^+ can combine with all available urinary buffers such as NH_3, phosphate, and bicarbonate or can remain as free H^+. The H^+ that combines with HCO_3^- forms CO_2, which diffuses back into the cells. The amount of free H^+ and H^+ bound to buffers is dependent on the amounts of the buffers present, the pK of the buffers, and the amount of H^+ secreted.

325. The answer is E. *(Ganong, 15/e. pp 669–671, 681–683. Rose, 3/e. pp 302–303.)* During chronic metabolic acidosis, the kidney attempts to restore body pH back to normal by increasing H^+ ion excretion and reabsorbing all the bicarbonate filtered at the glomerulus. Secretion of H^+ into the tubular lumen by the cells of both the proximal and distal nephron is enhanced. This enhances bicarbonate reabsorption in the proximal tubule and H^+ excretion in the distal nephron. During acidosis, the rate of production of ammonia from glutamine by the kidney is increased, which allows more H^+ to be excreted in the urine as NH_4^+. With the increase in acid excretion, the pH of the urine is decreased.

326. The answer is C. *(Berne, 2/e. pp 971–973. West, 12/e. pp 481–483, 496–497, 506.)* The primary renal effects of aldosterone are increased reabsorption of sodium and increased secretion of potassium and hydrogen. Aldosterone increases the permeability of the epithelial cells of the distal nephron to sodium and potassium and increases the number and activity of the active transport systems for these ions. Water reabsorption is increased as a consequence of the enhanced reabsorption of sodium. Excretion of ammonium and magnesium is increased by aldosterone.

327. The answer is C. *(Rose, 3/e. pp 211–215, 590–595. West, 12/e. pp 415–417.)* Sweat normally contains about 40 to 60 meq of sodium per liter of fluid. Thus, approximately 100 meq of sodium will be lost from the extracellular fluid during the exercise period, and when the lost water is replenished, the extracellular fluid will become hypotonic. The hypotonic extracellular fluid will equilibrate with the intracellular fluid and make it hypotonic as well. Because the extracellular fluid volume is dependent on the amount of sodium, the loss of sodium will result in a decreased extracellular fluid volume and an increased intracellular fluid volume after water is replaced.

328. The answer is C. *(Rose, 3/e. pp 299–304.)* Ammonia (NH_3) is produced from amino acids in the cells of the renal tubules (mainly the proximal tubules), and its rate of production increases during acidosis. This is important in acidosis because it increases the total amount of H^+ ion that can be excreted in a given volume of urine. The NH_3 freely diffuses into the tubular lumen, and because of the high pK_a (9.2) of the reaction, essentially all of it combines with H^+ to form NH_4^+. This maintains the driving force for more NH_3 to passively diffuse into the lumen. The NH_4^+ that is formed gets "trapped" in the tubules and excreted because the tubules are impermeable to this cation.

329. The answer is D. *(Rose, 3/e. pp 333–343. West, 12/e. pp 504–507.)* The amount of potassium excreted is controlled by the amount of potassium secreted by the distal tubule. Potassium secretion is a passive process that depends on the electrochemical gradient between the distal tubular cells and the tubular lumen and the permeability of the luminal cells to potassium. By inhibiting Na^+ reabsorption, the intraluminal potential becomes less negative and K^+ secretion is reduced. K^+-sparing diuretics such as amiloride act in this fashion. Aldosterone increases the intracellular potassium concentration by augmenting the activity of the Na-K pump and increasing the potassium permeability of the luminal membrane. Increasing dietary intake increases the plasma potassium concentration, which in turn stimulates aldosterone production. Although it is only a minor factor, increasing the rate of distal tubular flow increases secretion by maintaining a low potassium concentration within the filtrate and thus increasing the electrochemical gradient for potassium.

330. The answer is A. *(Berne, 2/e. pp 801–804, 811–813.)* An increase in arterial concentration of hydrogen ion from a normal value of 40 neq/L (pH 7.4) to 50 neq/L (pH 7.3) would constitute an acidosis. Acidosis in arterial blood rapidly stimulates the peripheral chemoreceptors in the carotid and aortic bodies. If the acidosis is a respiratory acidosis (elevated Pa_{CO_2}), the central chemoreceptors would be stimulated, but since the defect (hypoventilation) would be in the respiratory system, no respiratory compensation could occur. When Pa_{CO_2} is increased, plasma concentration of HCO_3^- is increased. Renal compensation for the acidosis causes a further increase in plasma concentration of HCO_3^-. If the acidosis is a metabolic acidosis, it takes time for the concentration of hydrogen ion in the brain's extracellular fluid to rise because of the presence of the blood-brain barrier. Therefore, the central chemoreceptors are stimulated only in chronic metabolic acidosis. Acidosis increases the formation of NH_3 in the kidney and increases the excretion of H^+ ions as ammonium (NH_4^+) ions. As more H^+ is excreted, the pH of the urine is decreased.

331. The answer is C. *(Rose, 3/e. pp 93–95, 127–130.)* Carbon dioxide and ammonia are lipid-soluble and thus able to cross all cell membranes. The ascending limb of the loop of Henle and, in the absence of ADH, the remainder of the distal nephron are impermeable to water. However, in the presence of ADH, water permeability of the distal nephron increases. The cortical and outer medullary collecting ducts are not permeable to urea, even in the presence of ADH.

332. The answer is B. *(West, 12/e. pp 436–438, 451–456.)* Sodium is isoosmotically reabsorbed from the proximal tubule; that is, when sodium is reabsorbed, water flows out of the proximal tubule to maintain a constant osmolarity. Thus, the concentration of sodium does not normally change as the filtrate flows through the proximal tubule. Since creatinine cannot be reabsorbed from the tubule, its concentration rises as water is reabsorbed. The concentrations of glucose, bicarbonate, and phosphate are all less at the end of the proximal tubule than at the beginning.

333. The answer is C. *(Rose, 3/e. pp 87, 122–131, 134.)* When a person is dehydrated, ADH secretion increases. In the presence of ADH, the distal nephron, distal convoluted tubule, and collecting duct become permeable to water and the filtrate within these portions of the nephron reaches osmotic equilibrium with the interstitial fluid surrounding them. The ascending limb of the loop of Henle is not affected by ADH and so remains impermeable to water. As sodium and other electrolytes are reabsorbed from the ascending limb, its filtrate becomes hypotonic. The glomerular filtrate and proximal tubular fluid remain isotonic to plasma, which in the case of dehydration is higher than normal.

334. The answer is C. *(West, 12/e. pp 462–463.)* In the ascending limb of the loop of Henle, sodium is actively transported by a transporter that has one binding site for sodium, one binding site for potassium, and two binding sites for chloride. Thus the transport of sodium is electrically neutral. Electrically neutral sodium transport also occurs in the distal convoluted tubule and connecting segment by a carrier that binds both sodium and chloride. In all other segments of the nephron, however, sodium transport is electrogenic; that is, sodium is transported unaccompanied by a negatively charged chloride ion.

335. The answer is B. *(Berne, 2/e. pp 803, 811–813. Rose, 3/e. pp 501–507.)* In diabetic ketoacidosis there is an increased production of acetoacetic and β-hydroxybutyric acids, which leads to an increase in plasma concentration of hydrogen ion. These fixed acids are buffered by all body buffers but mainly by bicarbonate. The concentration of plasma HCO_3^- is therefore below normal. The consumption of bicarbonate and the addition of the anions of the fixed acids to the plasma cause an elevation of the anion gap. The anion gap is equal to plasma $[Na^+]$ − (plasma $[HCO_3^-]$ + plasma $[Cl^-]$), and is normally about 12 to 15 meq/L. The acidosis would stimulate the carotid body chemoreceptors (and eventually the central chemoreceptors) to cause an increase in ventilation, which decreases arterial P_{CO_2}.

336. The answer is E. *(Berne, 2/e. pp 752–756.)* The fraction of plasma filtered out of the glomerular capillaries (FF) is proportional to the glomerular capillary pressure and the renal plasma flow (RPF). Decreasing the resistance of the afferent arteriole increases both the RPF and the glomerular capillary pressure; thus, FF will be increased. Since a larger fraction of a larger RPF is filtered, glomerular filtration rate will be increased. Because a larger fraction of fluid is removed from the plasma, the oncotic pressure of the plasma flowing into the peritubular capillaries will be increased.

337. The answer is C. *(Ganong, 15/e. p 672. Rose, 3/e. pp 97–98.)* When water is filtered across the glomerulus, the protein concentration (the oncotic pressure) within the capillaries increases, which in turn increases the efficiency by which water reabsorbed from the proximal tubule is returned to the circulatory system. If GFR increases, it results in a larger increase in oncotic pressure. This in turn increases the amount of water reabsorbed from the proximal tubule.

338. The answer is B. *(Berne, 2/e. pp 751–754. West, 12/e. pp 422–424.)* The glomerular filtration barrier through which solutes and water must pass to move from plasma to Bowman's capsule is composed of three layers: the capillary endothelium, the basement membrane, and the epithelium lining the nephron. The capillary endothelial cells contain fenestrations, or pores, which have a mean diameter of 70 nm. The epithelial cells lining the nephron are called *podocytes* because of numerous pedicles, or foot processes, that make contact with the basement membrane of the glomerular capillaries. The mesangium is located between the capillaries and the nephron. It contains mesangial cells surrounded by a matrix composed of a basement membrane–like material. Some mesangial cells are primarily involved in phagocytosis, while others are contractile and may influence glomerular blood flow. The macula densa is part of the juxtaglomerular apparatus and is outside the glomerulus.

339. The answer is E. *(Berne, 2/e. pp 785–787. Ganong, 15/e. pp 428–430.)* Juxtaglomerular (JG) cells are sensitive to changes in afferent arterial intraluminal pressure. Increased pressure within the afferent arteriole leads to a decrease in renin release, while decreased pressure tends to increase renin release. Angiotensin appears to inhibit renin release by initiating the flow of calcium into the JG cells. Renin release is increased in response to increased activity in the sympathetic neurons innervating the kidney. Prostaglandins, particularly PGI_2 and PGE_2, stimulate renin release. Stimulation of the macula densa leads to an increase in renin release, and although the mechanism is not fully understood, it appears that increased delivery of NaCl to the distal nephron is responsible for stimulating the macula densa. Aldosterone does not appear to have any direct effect on renin release.

340. The answer is C. *(Ganong, 15/e. pp 667–671. Rose, 3/e. pp 304–313.)* Filtered bicarbonate is reabsorbed in the kidney via an indirect mechanism that involves H^+ secretion into the lumen of the tubules. There, CO_2 is formed via the reaction $H^+ + HCO_3^- \rightarrow H_2CO_3 \rightarrow CO_2 + H_2O$. CO_2 freely diffuses into the cells, where in the presence of carbonic anhydrase the reaction reverses and forms H^+, which can again be secreted, and HCO_3^-, which exits the cells on the peritubular side and is thereby reabsorbed. Intracellular acidification of the renal tubular cells that occurs during hypercapnia and metabolic acidosis causes an increase in secretion of H^+ ion and therefore an increase in reabsorption of bicarbonate. Hyperkalemia causes intracellular alkalinization via exchange of K^+ for H^+ and therefore would decrease H^+ secretion and decrease HCO_3^- reabsorption. During volume depletion, there is an increase in the level of plasma aldosterone. Aldosterone stimulates H^+ secretion in the distal nephron, thereby increasing HCO_3^- reabsorption.

341. The answer is B. *(Rose, 3/e. pp 102–103. West, 12/e. pp 443, 457–458, 472–473.)* Most urea is synthesized in the liver. Its excretion is dependent on its concentration in plasma and the glomerular filtration rate (GFR) in the kidney. Approximately 50 to 60 percent of filtered plasma urea is passively reabsorbed in the proximal tubule at normal GFR. In renal insufficiency, in which GFR is decreased, filtrate remains in the tubules longer and more of the filtered urea is reabsorbed, which results in an increase in its plasma concentration. Urea is also passively reabsorbed in distal tubules and collecting ducts and recirculates back into tubular urine by means of the countercurrent mechanism.

342. The answer is B. *(Ganong, 15/e. pp 353–359. West, 12/e. pp 825–826, 830–831.)* Aldosterone binds to an intracellular receptor that causes an increased synthesis of a variety of proteins, including K^+ and Na^+ ion channels and Na-K ATPase, which together act to increase Na^+ reabsorption and K^+ secretion by the tubular cells of the distal nephron. H^+ secretion is also enhanced by aldosterone. Aldosterone secretion is stimulated by a decrease in blood volume (through the renin-angiotensin system) and by increased plasma K^+ concentrations. High blood pressure, if it has any effect on aldosterone, will cause a decrease in its secretion.

343. The answer is B. *(Berne, 2/e. pp 800–801. Rose, 3/e. pp 105–106, 183–184, 298–299.)* Phosphate in plasma is freely filtered at the glomerulus. The amount filtered is dependent on the plasma level of phosphate, which is directly influenced by the amount of phosphate in the diet. No phosphate is secreted into the lumen of the renal tubules; however, phosphate in the form HPO_4^{2-} can be reabsorbed. The level of parathyroid hormone (PTH) helps control the amount of HPO_4^{2-} reabsorption. An increase in the plasma PTH level decreases the renal reabsorption of phosphate. Phosphate in the form $H_2PO_4^-$, which is more abundant at low pH levels, is not reabsorbed. Therefore, when the pH of the urine is low and more phosphate is in the form $H_2PO_4^-$, less phosphate can be reabsorbed, and more H^+ will be excreted in the urine bound to phosphate. Phosphate is reabsorbed via a carrier-mediated process that exhibits a tubular maximum (Tm). If the Tm is decreased, maximum reabsorption would be reached at a lower plasma phosphate concentration and more phosphate would be excreted.

344. The answer is D. *(Berne, 2/e. pp 798–800. Ganong, 15/e. pp 457–458. Rose, 3/e. pp 295–297.)* Carbonic anhydrase is the enzyme that catalyzes the following reaction: $CO_2 + H_2O \overset{C.A.}{\rightleftharpoons} H_2CO_3 \rightleftharpoons H^+ + HCO_3^-$. In the nephron it is located within tubular cells of both the proximal tubule and distal nephron (i.e., distal tubule, collecting tubule, and collecting duct), where it provides H^+ for secretion into the lumen and HCO_3^- for transport across the basolateral surfaces of the tubular cells. It is also located extracellularly on the brush border of the luminal surface of the cells of the proximal tubule S_1 and S_2 segments but is generally not located on the luminal surface of the cells of the distal nephron. In the proximal tubule, this luminal carbonic anhydrase catalyzes the formation of CO_2 and H_2O from H_2CO_3, which is in turn formed from filtered HCO_3^- and H^+ secreted into the lumen by the Na^+/H^+ exchanger of the cells of the proximal tubule. The CO_2 formed diffuses into the cells, where it can again form H^+ and HCO_3^- for secretion and reabsorption, respectively. The parietal cells of the gastric mucosa actively secrete HCl into the stomach cavity. The H^+ secreted and the HCO_3^- that is transported across the basolateral membrane of the cells are formed from the hydration of CO_2, catalyzed by the carbonic anhydrase within the parietal cells.

345. The answer is A. *(Berne, 2/e. pp 787–788. Rose, 3/e. pp 157–159.)* The principal physiologic action of antidiuretic hormone (ADH) is to increase water retention by the kidney. The hormone acts on the distal nephron to increase its permeability so that water more readily enters the hypertonic interstitium of the renal pyramids. Thus, the concentration of solutes in the urine is increased. ADH increases Na^+ reabsorption so that the actual amount of Na^+ excreted is decreased. It also acts as a vasoconstrictor; hence, it is called *arginine vasopressin (AVP)*. ADH has no effect on glomerular filtration rate, and because it increases water reabsorption, it would decrease urine formation.

346. The answer is D. *(Ganong, 15/e. pp 671–673. West, 12/e. pp 480–485.)* Sodium reabsorption in the distal tubule is primarily regulated by aldosterone. Increases in aldosterone increase Na^+ reabsorption. Antidiuretic hormone will increase Na^+ reabsorption by the collecting ducts. Neither sympathetic nerve stimulation nor angiotensin has a direct effect on the distal tubule, but both increase Na^+ reabsorption by the proximal tubule. Atrial natriuretic hormone (ANH, or ANP) increases Na^+ excretion.

347. The answer is E. *(Berne, 2/e. pp 804–805, 808–813.)* When fixed acid is added to the body, all defense mechanisms against a change in body pH are used. Buffering is the first line of defense. The extracellular fluid buffers (especially bicarbonate) and blood buffers (especially hemoglobin) would "see" the acid load first. Gradually the H^+ would move into cells, where the intracellular buffers would participate in buffering. With a decrease in plasma pH the kidneys would begin to excrete excess H^+ ions and make "new" bicarbonate to replace that lost in the buffering process. Although the decrease in body pH caused by the acid load would be combated by the body buffers, no buffer is perfect and there would still be a decrease in pH. This would stimulate the carotid body chemoreceptors and ventilation would increase to lower the P_{CO_2} and raise the body pH to further combat the acid load.

348. The answer is B. *(Berne, 2/e. pp 787–791. West, 12/e. pp 470–476.)* The counter-current multiplier concentrates urine by establishing a medullary interstitium that is hypertonic to plasma. In the presence of ADH, the fluid in the collecting duct reaches osmotic equilibrium with the medullary interstitium and thus is excreted as a hypertonic fluid. Anything that reduces the medullary hypertonicity, such as increasing the flow of filtrate through the loop of Henle or decreasing the activity of the Na-K pump, will decrease the ability of the kidney to excrete a concentrated urine. If the permeability of the collecting duct to water is decreased, the urine's tonicity will be decreased.

349. The answer is D. *(West, 12/e. pp 429–434.)* The amount of fluid filtered by the glomerulus (the GFR) will increase if filtration pressure rises or plasma oncotic pressure decreases. A decrease in filtration will occur if the pressure within the kidney rises. Intrarenal pressure will increase if the urine is unable to flow through the urethra and backs up into the kidney. The kidney uses a variety of regulatory mechanisms to keep GFR constant when there is a change in renal perfusion pressure. For example, if an increase in circulating blood volume causes an increase in perfusion pressure, the afferent arteriole will constrict to keep renal blood flow and GFR at their normal levels. However, if the afferent arteriolar resistance increases without an increase in perfusion pressure, the pressure within the glomerulus will decrease and cause a decrease in GFR. A similar result will occur if the efferent arteriolar resistance falls.

350. The answer is C. *(Berne, 2/e. pp 787–789. West, 12/e. pp 464–469.)* The filtrate remains isotonic as it passes through the proximal tubule and so it enters the loop of Henle as an isotonic fluid. As the filtrate flows through the descending limb of the loop of Henle, its tonicity increases as Na^+ enters and water leaves the filtrate. Na^+ is reabsorbed from the ascending limb, but because the ascending limb is impermeable to water, water does not follow and the filtrate leaving the loop of Henle becomes hypotonic to plasma. In the presence of ADH, the filtrate reaches isotonicity with the surrounding interstitium, which is isotonic to plasma in the cortex and hypertonic in the medulla. Thus, as the fluid passes into the cortical collecting duct, it is isotonic to plasma, and when it passes through the medullary collecting duct, it becomes hypertonic to plasma.

351–352. The answers are: 351-E, 352-A. *(Ganong, 15/e. pp 680–686. Guyton, 8/e. pp 340–343.)* Acid-base disturbances fall into four major groups that can be separated by examining their effects on the body's major buffer system—HCO_3^-/CO_2. Disturbances influencing one of these buffer substances will alter their ratio and alter pH.

Metabolic acidosis may result from (1) overproduction of organic acids such as acetoacetic acid in diabetes mellitus or lactic acid in hypoxia, (2) decreased renal excretion, or (3) drug ingestion. This increase in nonvolatile acid is neutralized by bicarbonate so that the net result is a decrease in bicarbonate without a change in P_{CO_2} (point E in the graph accompanying the question). Subsequent respiratory compensation would lower P_{CO_2}. In situations involving excess bicarbonate ingestion or acid loss (vomiting), the concentration of plasma HCO_3^- increases with no change in P_{CO_2}, and this produces metabolic alkalosis (point B). Subsequent respiratory compensation could cause a slight rise in P_{CO_2}.

Respiratory acidosis results from an increase in P_{CO_2}, which can be caused by primary pulmonary disease or any mechanism that compromises respiratory function and leads to CO_2 retention. In this condition, P_{CO_2} is increased with no acute change in concentration of HCO_3^- (point D). Hyperventilation, whether caused by voluntary action, exposure to altitude, or by disease of the central nervous system, promotes loss of CO_2 and lowers P_{CO_2}, with resultant respiratory alkalosis (point A).

The occurrence of each of these processes induces a compensatory response that attempts to restore the arterial pH to normal. In chronic respiratory acidosis, the kidney excretes hydrogen ion and acts to increase the plasma bicarbonate level to return the pH toward or to normal (point C). Arterial P_{CO_2} remains elevated. In many clinical situations, multiple acid-base disturbances may occur.

353–357. The answers are: 353-C, 354-D, 355-A, 356-E, 357-A. *(Ganong, 15/e. pp 627–628, 680–686.)* In metabolic acidosis (point C) there is an increase in the amount of fixed acids in the blood. This decreases arterial pH to a value lower than the normal value of 7.4 (point B). The low arterial pH stimulates carotid body chemoreceptors to increase ventilation, which results in a reduction of the arterial P_{CO_2} level below the normal value of about 40 mmHg (hyperventilation). In metabolic alkalosis the arterial pH is elevated but the arterial P_{CO_2} is usually normal or only slightly elevated. In acute respiratory acidosis (point D), the primary disturbance is an increase in arterial P_{CO_2}, which results in a decrease in arterial pH. If the condition persists, the kidneys act to compensate by excreting hydrogen ions and increasing the plasma bicarbonate level. This brings the arterial pH back toward or even to normal, while the arterial P_{CO_2} remains elevated (chronic respiratory acidosis, point E). In acute respiratory alkalosis (point A), the primary disturbance is a decrease in the arterial P_{CO_2} level. An example of this condition is the hyperventilation that occurs upon ascent to altitude. At altitude, the reduction in arterial P_{O_2} that occurs as a result of the reduced barometric pressure stimulates the carotid body chemoreceptors to increase alveolar ventilation. In acute respiratory alkalosis arterial pH is elevated because of the reduction in arterial P_{CO_2}. With time, the kidneys act to excrete bicarbonate ion, which brings the arterial pH back toward normal. The arterial P_{CO_2} remains low.

358–362. The answers are: 358-C, 359-H, 360-E, 361-C, 362-B. *(Berne, 2/e. pp 751–752, 763–764, 769–770, 787–789. West, 12/e. pp 425–426, 433–434, 456, 466–467, 481–482.)* In the proximal tubule, sodium diffuses passively across the luminal membrane of the epithelial cells and is then actively pumped out of the cell by an Na-K pump located on the basolateral surface. The presence of sodium in the basolateral spaces establishes an osmotic gradient, which causes water to flow out of the lumen. The flow of water down this osmotic gradient maintains the isotonicity of the filtrate and the reabsorbed fluid.

Antidiuretic hormone (ADH) regulates the osmolarity of the extracellular fluid by varying the permeability of the collecting duct to water. The increase in permeability to water caused by ADH allows water to flow out of the collecting duct down an osmotic gradient between the lumen and the medullary interstitium.

The high osmolarity of the medullary interstitium is created by the countercurrent multiplication system of the loop of Henle. The active transport process responsible for the countercurrent multiplier (a carrier that transports one ion of Na^+, one ion of K^+, and two ions of Cl^-) is located on the thick portion of the ascending limb of the loop of Henle.

PTH regulates the extracellular concentration of calcium and phosphate ions. In the kidney, it binds to a receptor on the basolateral surface of the epithelial cells of the proximal tubule and causes a decrease in reabsorption of phosphate.

The proximal tubule is the site of reabsorption of glucose (via secondary active transport). Glucose enters the tubular cells on a carrier that also binds sodium. The sodium that enters is then pumped out of the cell on the basolateral side by Na,K-ATPase.

The path of blood flow at the level of the nephron is first through the afferent arteriole and then through the glomerulus, which is composed of a capillary tuft found only in the cortex of the kidney. Blood from the glomerulus flows through the efferent arteriole into the peritubular capillaries. The vasa rectae are a capillary network found in the medulla of the kidney in association with the loop of Henle. They help to maintain the high medullary interstitial osmolarity established by the countercurrent multiplication system.

The smooth muscle of the afferent arteriole is the site of myogenic autoregulation of renal blood flow. An increase in blood pressure causes a constriction of the afferent arteriole. The aim of this mechanism is to maintain renal blood flow and glomerular filtration at constant rates.

The afferent arteriole in apposition to the beginning of the distal tubule forms the juxtaglomerular apparatus (JGA). This consists of the macula densa, which is composed of specialized cells of the distal tubule, and the juxtaglomerular (or granular) cells, which are specialized cells of the walls of the afferent arteriole. In the juxtaglomerular cells are granules containing the enzyme renin, which, when released into the blood, converts angiotensinogen (renin substrate) to angiotensin I.

Aldosterone is a hormone released by the zona glomerulosa of the adrenal cortex. An increase in aldosterone causes an increase in the reabsorption of sodium by the cells of the collecting duct by increasing sodium entry into the cells. The sodium is then pumped out via the Na,K-ATPase.

Gastrointestinal System

DIRECTIONS: Each question below contains five suggested responses. Select the **one best** response to each question.

363. Saliva has all the following constituents EXCEPT

(A) bicarbonate
(B) phosphate
(C) chloride
(D) glucose
(E) lysozyme

364. All the following are correct statements about pancreatic exocrine secretion EXCEPT

(A) bicarbonate-rich fluid is secreted by ductal epithelial cells in response to secretin
(B) secretion of enzymes by acinar cells occurs in response to cholecystokinin
(C) vagotomy augments secretion of enzymes after a meal
(D) secretin and cholecystokinin both act via formation of cyclic nucleotide second messengers
(E) gastrin stimulates both enzyme and bicarbonate secretion

365. Peristaltic waves in the small intestine are characterized by which of the following statements?

(A) They are controlled primarily by extrinsic innervation
(B) They involve simultaneous contraction of the circular and longitudinal muscles
(C) They occur in response to distention of the wall
(D) They are preceded by increased fluid secretion by the intestinal mucosa
(E) None of the above

366. All the following statements about bile acids are correct EXCEPT

(A) bile acids are secreted as conjugated bile salts by the liver
(B) bile acids are dehydroxylated by intestinal bacteria
(C) bile acids are absorbed in the intestine and return to the liver via the portal vein
(D) bile acids facilitate absorption of fat by emulsifying glycerides
(E) sulfation of bile acids promotes their uptake in the intestine

367. Chronic administration of antacids and maintenance of a gastric pH that is about 7 would cause gastrin levels to

(A) decrease
(B) increase
(C) decrease, then subsequently increase
(D) increase, then decrease
(E) remain unchanged

368. Which phase of secretion of acid will be most affected by a vagotomy?

(A) Basal
(B) Cephalic
(C) Gastric
(D) Interdigestive
(E) Intestinal

369. Which one of the following processes applies to the proximal stomach?

(A) Accommodation
(B) Peristalsis
(C) Retropulsion
(D) Segmentation
(E) Trituration

370. After secretion of trypsinogen into the duodenum, the enzyme is converted into its active form, trypsin, by

(A) enteropeptidase
(B) procarboxypeptidase
(C) pancreatic lipase
(D) previously secreted trypsin
(E) an alkaline pH

371. The major mechanism for absorption of sodium from the small intestine is

(A) nonelectrolytic cotransport
(B) cotransport with potassium
(C) electrogenic transport
(D) neutral NaCl absorption
(E) solvent drag

372. The presence of chyme within the small intestine will lead to all the following EXCEPT

(A) a decrease in the rate of gastric emptying
(B) an increase in the secretion of gastric acid
(C) an increase in intestinal segmentation
(D) contraction of the gallbladder
(E) pancreatic secretion of bicarbonate

373. Pharmacologic blockade of histamine H_2 receptors in the gastric mucosa

(A) inhibits both gastrin-induced and vagally mediated secretion of acid
(B) inhibits gastrin-induced but not vagally mediated secretion of acid
(C) has no effect on either gastrin-induced or vagally mediated secretion of acid
(D) prevents activation of adenyl cyclase by gastrin
(E) causes an increase in potassium transport by gastric parietal (oxyntic) cells

374. Bile salts promote absorption of lipids as a result of their ability to do all the following EXCEPT

(A) form micelles, or water-soluble complexes
(B) reduce surface tension of fat particles
(C) increase transit time of lipids in the gut
(D) emulsify fat
(E) stimulate reesterification in the mucosal cells

375. The emptying rate of the stomach is regulated by hormonal and neural mechanisms that respond to both chemical and mechanical stimuli. The rate of gastric emptying is influenced by all the following factors EXCEPT

(A) carbohydrate in gastric contents
(B) secretion of gastrin by antral G cells
(C) distention of the duodenum
(D) osmolarity of duodenal contents
(E) acidity of chyme entering the duodenum

376. Gallbladder contraction is controlled primarily by the hormone

(A) enterogastrone
(B) cholecystokinin-pancreozymin (CCK)
(C) insulin
(D) secretin
(E) glucagon

377. Mass movements (strong peristalsis) in the colon would be abolished by

(A) vagotomy
(B) extrinsic denervation
(C) distention of the colon
(D) destruction of Meissner's plexus
(E) destruction of Auerbach's plexus

378. Dietary fat is absorbed chiefly in the

(A) stomach
(B) jejunum
(C) ileum
(D) cecum
(E) ascending colon

379. Dietary fat, after being processed, is extruded from the mucosal cells of the gastrointestinal tract into the lymphatic ducts in the form of

(A) monoglycerides
(B) diglycerides
(C) triglycerides
(D) chylomicrons
(E) free fatty acids

380. Insulin produces all the following effects EXCEPT

(A) increased utilization of glucose
(B) increased lipolysis
(C) decreased proteolysis
(D) decreased gluconeogenesis
(E) decreased ketogenesis

381. Acute obstruction of the common bile duct produced experimentally will incur which of the following changes in plasma and urinary levels of bilirubin?

	Unconjugated Bilirubin in Plasma	Conjugated Bilirubin in Plasma	Conjugated Bilirubin in Urine
(A)	Increase	No change	Increase
(B)	No change	Increase	Increase
(C)	Decrease	Decrease	Decrease
(D)	Increase	Decrease	Increase
(E)	Decrease	No change	Increase

382. The gastrointestinal tract, from the esophagus to intestine, is innervated by the intramural nerve plexus. Stimulation of the myenteric plexus increases all the following EXCEPT the

(A) tonic contractions (tone) of the gut wall
(B) intensity of rhythmic contractions
(C) rate of rhythmic contractions
(D) velocity of excitatory waves along the gut wall
(E) rate of production of epithelial cells lining the gut

383. Absorption of fat involves all the following processes EXCEPT

(A) acylation of glycerol-3-phosphate
(B) acylation of mono- and diglycerides
(C) thioesterification of fatty acids
(D) hydrolysis of luminal fat by pancreatic lipase
(E) acidification of luminal contents prior to emulsification

384. The pancreas has both an endocrine and an exocrine function. The nonhormonal substances released by the pancreas serve all the following functions EXCEPT

(A) neutralizing the acid that enters the duodenum
(B) breaking down carbohydrate bonds
(C) breaking down lipids
(D) breaking down proteins
(E) increasing trypsin activity

385. All the following statements concerning normal human pancreatic juice are true EXCEPT

(A) its pH is approximately 8.0
(B) it has a high bicarbonate content
(C) over 1000 mL are secreted per day
(D) it contains cholesterol esterase
(E) its secretion is primarily under neural control

386. Secretion of gastric acid can be stimulated by which of the following?

(A) Administration of cimetidine
(B) Methylation of histamine
(C) Parasympathetic stimulation
(D) Release of somatostatin
(E) None of the above

387. Gas within the colon is primarily derived from which one of the following sources?

(A) CO_2 liberated by the interaction of HCO_3^- and H^+
(B) Diffusion from the blood
(C) Fermentation of undigested oligosaccharides by bacteria
(D) Swallowed atmospheric air
(E) None of the above

388. Removal of the antrum is associated with

(A) a decrease in gastric compliance
(B) an increase in maximal output of acid
(C) an increase in basal output of acid
(D) an increase in the rate of gastric emptying of solids
(E) an increase in the serum gastrin level

389. Removal of the terminal ileum will result in

(A) a decrease in absorption of amino acids
(B) an increase in the water content of the feces
(C) an increase in the concentration of bile acid in the enterohepatic circulation
(D) a decrease in the fat content of the feces
(E) an increase in the absorption of iron

390. Vitamins synthesized by intestinal bacteria and absorbed in significant quantities include

(A) vitamin B_6
(B) vitamin K
(C) thiamine
(D) riboflavin
(E) folic acid

391. Secretion of acid by the gastric mucosa is correctly described by which one of the following statements?

(A) It is carried out by chief cells
(B) It is inhibited by acetylcholine
(C) It is inhibited by antihistamines taken by allergy patients
(D) It involves active transport of H^+
(E) It involves release of HCl from zymogen granules

392. Gastric inhibitory peptide is correctly described by all the following statements EXCEPT

(A) it is secreted by cells in the antrum of the stomach
(B) its secretion is enhanced by oral administration of glucose
(C) its secretion is inhibited by somatostatin
(D) it increases insulin secretion
(E) it decreases gastric motility

393. Which one of the following statements about the colon is correct?

(A) Absorption of Na^+ in the colon is under hormonal (aldosterone) control
(B) Bile acids enhance absorption of water from the colon
(C) Net absorption of HCO_3^- occurs in the colon
(D) Net absorption of K^+ occurs in the colon
(E) The luminal potential in the colon is positive

394. Excess fluid loss in the stool (diarrhea) can develop as a consequence of all the following EXCEPT

(A) a decrease in neutral NaCl absorption
(B) bile salts in the colon
(C) fatty acids in the colon
(D) an accumulation of nonabsorbable sugars in the small intestine
(E) a decrease in colonic motility

395. Gastric acid secretion is stimulated by the presence of all the following EXCEPT

(A) acetylcholine
(B) caffeine
(C) gastrin
(D) histamine
(E) norepinephrine

396. The intestinal brush border promotes digestion by all the following EXCEPT

(A) acting as a protective barrier for intestinal epithelium
(B) facilitating movement of intestinal contents
(C) increasing the surface area of the intestinal mucosa
(D) supplying digestive enzymes
(E) supplying specialized transport systems

397. All the following statements about migrating motor complexes (MMCs) in humans are correct EXCEPT

(A) they are correlated with increases in plasma motilin
(B) they are periods of intense contractile activity
(C) they occur only during the interdigestive period
(D) they occur exclusively in the small intestine
(E) they require an intact intrinsic nervous system for coordinated propagation

398. The stimulation of release of pancreatic secretions normally involves all the following EXCEPT

(A) acetylcholine
(B) cholecystokinin
(C) histamine
(D) neural stimulation
(E) secretin

399. Contraction of the gallbladder is correctly described by which one of the following statements?

(A) It is inhibited by a fat-rich meal
(B) It is inhibited by the presence of amino acids in the duodenum
(C) It is stimulated by atropine
(D) It occurs in response to cholecystokinin
(E) It occurs simultaneously with the contraction of the sphincter of Oddi

400. In a normal person, all the following circumstances will elicit the enterogastric reflex EXCEPT

(A) increased duodenal pressure
(B) irritation of the small bowel
(C) excessive protein catabolites in the duodenum
(D) acid chyme in the duodenum
(E) pancreatic juice in the duodenum

401. Acidification of the duodenum will

(A) decrease pancreatic secretion of bicarbonate
(B) increase secretion of gastric acid
(C) decrease gastric emptying
(D) increase contraction of the gallbladder
(E) increase contraction of the sphincter of Oddi

402. True statements about bile acids include all the following EXCEPT

(A) conjugation of bile acids with glycine or taurine increases the likelihood of formation of micelles
(B) dihydroxy bile acids decrease the absorption of water from the colon
(C) primary bile acids are formed in the liver from cholesterol
(D) secondary bile acids are formed in the small bowel
(E) secretin increases the rate of synthesis of primary bile acids by the liver

403. An important function of the gastric mucosa is secretion of

(A) cholecystokinin
(B) enteropeptidase
(C) intrinsic factor
(D) secretin
(E) trypsinogen

404. Which one of the following is a true statement about the lower esophageal sphincter?

(A) It is a smooth muscle band similar to the pylorus in thickness
(B) Its resting tension is decreased in achalasia
(C) Its resting tension is increased during pregnancy
(D) It does not respond to sympathetic stimulation
(E) It relaxes during swallowing

405. Which of the following is a paracrine secretion?

(A) Cholecystokinin
(B) Gastrin
(C) Histamine
(D) Secretin
(E) None of the above

406. Intestinal proteolysis is accomplished by all the following EXCEPT

(A) carboxypeptidase
(B) chymotrypsin
(C) elastase
(D) pepsin
(E) trypsin

407. Human bile acids include all the following substances EXCEPT

(A) cholic acid
(B) chenodeoxycholic acid
(C) deoxycholic acid
(D) lithocholic acid
(E) uric acid

408. In contrast to secondary esophageal peristalsis, primary esophageal peristalsis is characterized by which of the following statements?

(A) It does not involve relaxation of the lower esophageal sphincter
(B) It involves contraction of esophageal smooth muscle
(C) It is not influenced by the intrinsic nervous system
(D) It has an oropharyngeal phase
(E) None of the above

409. Absorption of fat-soluble vitamins requires

(A) intrinsic factor
(B) chymotrypsin
(C) pancreatic lipase
(D) pancreatic amylase
(E) none of the above

410. The concept that active transport is the mechanism for absorption of monosaccharides in the gut is supported by all the following statements EXCEPT

(A) transport can be blocked by metabolic inhibitors
(B) transport is selective for different sugars
(C) a maximum rate of transport exists for individual monosaccharides
(D) competition exists among sugars for the carrier mechanism
(E) transport can occur bidirectionally

Gastrointestinal System
Answers

363. The answer is D. *(West, 12/e. pp 647–650.)* Glucose is not normally found in saliva; even in diabetic patients, none or only a small amount is found. Lysozyme is a salivary enzyme that can lyse certain bacteria, including *Staphylococcus, Proteus,* and *Streptococcus.* Bicarbonate is present in saliva; its concentration increases with salivary flow. Chloride is also normally present, and its concentration may vary with salivary flow. The concentration of phosphate is relatively independent of the rate of salivary flow.

364. The answer is C. *(Guyton, 8/e. pp 718–720.)* Cholecystokinin released in response to the presence of amino acids and peptides in the duodenum is the major stimulant of enzyme secretion by pancreatic acinar cells and also weakly stimulates secretion of bicarbonate-rich fluid by ductal epithelial cells. Parasympathetic stimulation via the vagus is also a major stimulant of enzyme secretion. Thus, vagotomy drastically reduces enzyme secretion after a meal. The major stimulant for bicarbonate secretion is secretin, which is released from the duodenum in response to acidification of the luminal contents. Both cholecystokinin and secretin act by stimulating the formation of cyclic nucleotide second messengers—cyclic AMP in the case of secretin and cyclic GMP in the case of cholecystokinin. Gastrin can mimic the effects of cholecystokinin because both have the same C terminal amino acid sequence.

365. The answer is C. *(West, 12/e. pp 635–638.)* Peristalsis in the small intestine occurs in response to distention of the intestinal wall and is mediated primarily by the intramural myenteric plexus, which may be influenced by its extrinsic innervation. It consists of a compound wave of contraction and relaxation in which the longitudinal muscle contracts first; this is followed by contraction of circular muscle, which occurs 90 degrees out of phase. Secretion of intestinal fluid usually accompanies or follows the peristaltic wave and aids in the dilution and lubrication of the chyme as it passes.

366. The answer is E. *(Guyton, 8/e. pp 720–723.)* Primary bile acids are synthesized from cholesterol in the liver by the addition of hydroxyl and carboxyl groups and are secreted as amide conjugates with either taurine or glycine. Dehydroxylation of these compounds by intestinal bacteria forms secondary bile acids. Both primary and secondary bile acids are reabsorbed primarily by active transport in the ileum and return to the liver via the portal vein, where they are reutilized and secreted in the bile. Because they possess both hydrophobic and hydrophilic properties, bile acids and their salts accumulate at lipid-water interfaces and thus emulsify dietary fat and promote its hydrolysis. Sulfation of bile acids occurs in the liver. Since sulfated bile acids are not reabsorbed in the ileum, this process is a major route for excretion of these compounds in the feces.

367. The answer is B. *(Guyton, 8/e. pp 715–716.)* Secretion of gastrin by antral G cells occurs in response to antral distention and certain chemical stimuli, such as amino acids and calcium, but is directly inhibited by the presence of hydrochloric acid in the antrum. This feedback inhibition is important in protecting the gastric mucosa from excessive acid and also in maintaining optimum pH for function of gastric enzymes. Chronic administration of antacid to maintain gastric pH at 7 would abolish this negative feedback control mechanism and thus cause an increase in gastrin secretion.

368. The answer is B. *(Berne, 2/e. pp 698–700.)* Secretion of acid occurs because of the complex interaction of neural, hormonal, and paracrine stimuli. The predominant excitatory neural input occurs via the vagus nerve. When vagal input is removed, secretion of acid is decreased. Because the cephalic phase of secretion of acid is mediated exclusively by the vagus nerve, it will be the most affected by vagotomy. Secretion of acid will continue during the other phases (although it will be reduced) because of the other pathways for stimulation.

369. The answer is A. *(Berne, 2/e. pp 665–666, 672–674.)* Increases in intragastric volume normally are not associated with large increases in intragastric pressure because of distention-mediated activation of a vagovagal inhibitory reflex, the accommodation reflex. The reflex is a property of the proximal stomach only and counterbalances the stretch-induced myogenic contraction of the gastric smooth muscle. *Peristalsis, trituration* (grinding), and *retropulsion* (mixing) are terms referring to the contractile activity and functions of the distal stomach. Segmentation is the primary contractile pattern of the small intestine during the digestive period.

370. The answer is A. *(Guyton, 8/e. p 718.)* Liberation of the enzyme enteropeptidase (enterokinase) from the duodenal mucosal cells causes the inactive trypsinogen to be converted to the active form, trypsin. Enteropeptidase contains 41 percent polysaccharide. It is this high level of polysaccharide that is responsible for the fact that enteropeptidase itself is not digested. Trypsin is responsible for the conversion of chymotrypsinogens and other proenzymes into their active forms.

371. The answer is D. *(Berne, 2/e. pp 724–728.)* Absorption of sodium is the primary absorptive event in the small intestine. Absorption of Na^+ is necessary for absorption of water and other electrolytes. Although multiple pathways exist for the absorption of Na^+, neutral absorption is the major mechanism. Neutral absorption may occur in two ways: Na^+ cotransported with Cl^- or in exchange for H^+ ions.

372. The answer is B. *(Berne, 2/e. pp 669–671, 674–675, 699–701.)* Food in the small intestine elicits a number of neurally and hormonally mediated reflexes that govern the activity of the GI tract. Cholecystokinin (CCK) and secretin act to stimulate secretion of pancreatic enzymes and HCO_3^-, while at the same time they play a role in the inhibitory feedback regulation of gastric emptying and secretion of acid. The distention caused by the presence of food activates a complex series of reflexes mediated by the intrinsic nervous system; these reflexes increase the segmental contractile pattern of the bowel.

373. The answer is A. *(Ganong, 15/e. pp 456–458. Guyton, 8/e. pp 715–716.)* Secretion of acid by gastric parietal (oxyntic) cells involves stimulation of adenyl cyclase and cyclic AMP–mediated stimulation of the active transport of chloride and potassium-hydrogen ion exchange. Neither gastrin nor vagal stimulation activates adenyl cyclase directly; both depend on concomitant release of histamine and histamine-induced activation of adenyl cyclase. Blockade of histamine H_2 receptors by drugs such as cimetidine thus inhibits both gastrin-induced and vagally mediated secretion of acid.

374. The answer is C. *(Ganong, 15/e. pp 464–467. Guyton, 8/e. pp 722–723.)* Bile salts combine with lipids to form micelles. Micelles are water-soluble complexes that are more easily absorbed than uncombined lipids, which are hydrophobic. Prior to micelle formation, bile salts exercise an emulsifying action on fat particles that involves a reduction in surface tension of such particles. Emulsification of fat particles, in which fatty acids and glycerides also participate, facilitates digestion and absorption. Reesterification of fatty acids in the mucosal cells—another prerequisite for absorption—also is stimulated by bile salts.

375. The answer is A. *(Guyton, 8/e. pp 702–703.)* The rate of gastric emptying is regulated by stimuli that originate in both the stomach and duodenum and that are coordinated to prevent movement of gastric contents at a rate faster than they can be processed by the small bowel. Distention of the duodenum, increased concentration of hydrogen ion, and inappropriate osmolarity all will retard gastric emptying. Gastrin, however, enhances gastric motility and promotes gastric emptying. Carbohydrate is rapidly hydrolyzed and absorbed and has little effect on the rate of gastric emptying.

376. The answer is B. *(Guyton, 8/e. p 722.)* Although several intestinal hormones, including gastrin, cause contraction of the gallbladder, the principal mechanism involved is stimulation by the hormone cholecystokinin-pancreozymin (CCK). CCK is elaborated in the duodenum in response to food. It supplements the action of secretin to produce alkaline pancreatic juice and retards gastric emptying. CCK is also thought to be associated with secretin in promoting contraction of the pyloric sphincter.

377. The answer is E. *(Guyton, 8/e. pp 705–707.)* Mass movements (strong peristalsis) in the colon occur about two to three times per day. They are initiated and continued by Auerbach's plexus and are independent of any extrinsic forces or innervation. At least three mass movements are usually required for the colonic contents to reach the rectum. Meissner's plexus is submucosal and has a principally sensory function.

378. The answer is B. *(Ganong, 15/e. p 443.)* Although a certain amount of dietary fat is absorbed in the ileum, the greatest portion is absorbed in the upper portion of the small intestine, mainly in the duodenum and jejunum. From the normal diet, 95 percent of ingested fat is absorbed. Feces contain about 5 percent fat, which is in part derived from cellular debris and microorganisms.

379. The answer is D. *(Ganong, 15/e. p 443.)* Triglycerides are hydrolyzed to monoglycerides and taken into mucosal cells. If the fatty acids are short chains (less than 10 to 12 carbon atoms), they are extruded in the form of free fatty acids into the portal blood. If the fatty acids are long chains, they are extruded in the form of chylomicrons into the lymphatic system. Chylomicrons represent triglycerides and esters of cholesterol that have been invested in the intestinal mucosa with a coating of phospholipid, protein, and cholesterol.

380. The answer is B. *(Ganong, 15/e. pp 315–317.)* The main function of insulin is to stimulate anabolic reactions involving carbohydrates, fats, proteins, and nucleic acids. Therefore, insulin increases the utilization of glucose while stimulating lipogenesis and proteogenesis. By promoting utilization of glucose in cells, insulin diminishes the need for gluconeogenesis and ketogenesis.

381. The answer is B. *(West, 12/e. pp 682–684.)* Unconjugated bilirubin, which is a breakdown product of the heme ring of hemoglobin, is taken up from plasma by the liver, conjugated with glucuronic acid, and released via the bile duct into the gastrointestinal tract. Under normal conditions, some conjugated bilirubin is reabsorbed by the intestine. The kidney clears only conjugated bilirubin. Thus, acute obstruction of the bile duct does not affect the rate of hepatic conjugation of bilirubin but does result in a "backup" of conjugated bilirubin in plasma and in its eventual clearance by the kidney.

382. The answer is E. *(Guyton, 8/e. pp 690–691.)* The intramural nerve plexus of the gastrointestinal tract consists of two groups of neurons: (1) the myenteric (Auerbach's) plexus located between the muscular layers and (2) the submucosal (Meissner's) plexus. Stimulation of the intramural nerve plexus increases motor activity of the intestine, which is reflected in increased muscle tone as well as in an increase in the velocity and intensity of the rhythmic contractions that propel luminal contents. Replacement of epithelial cells lining the gut occurs at a constant rate and is not controlled by the myenteric plexus. As surface epithelium is shed, cells deep in the crypts proliferate to maintain the lining.

383. The answer is E. *(Ganong, 15/e. pp 442–443.)* Absorption of fat occurs primarily in the duodenum and proximal jejunum and initially involves the formation of micelles by bile salts and phospholipids, fatty acids, and glycerides in order to solubilize the water-insoluble fat. Micelle formation is enhanced by the alkalinization of luminal contents by pancreatic and biliary secretions, a process that favors dissociation of fatty acids and improves their water solubility and interactions with other micellar components. Pancreatic lipase acts on micelles, releasing fatty acids and 2-monoglycerides that are taken up into mucosal cells. Fatty acids are then activated to acyl CoA thioesters and incorporated into phospholipids and triglycerides. They are released into the lymph as chylomicrons.

384. The answer is E. *(Guyton, 8/e. pp 718–719.)* The pancreas releases several enzymes that aid in the digestion of fat, protein, and carbohydrate and that demonstrate optimal activity above pH 7.0. Pancreatic secretions are rich in HCO_3^- and thus neutralize acid entering the duodenum. Trypsin is a proteolytic enzyme that is released in the intestinal lumen from its inactive precursor, trypsinogen, which is formed in the pancreas. Activation of trypsin within the pancreas is prevented by the pancreatic secretion of a trypsin inhibitor, which, by blocking the activation of trypsin, prevents autodigestion.

385. The answer is E. *(Ganong, 15/e. pp 462–464. Guyton, 8/e. pp 718–719.)* Pancreatic juice is rich in bicarbonate and, having a pH of about 8.0, neutralizes gastric acid entering the duodenum. It is secreted at the rate of 1 to 2 L per day and contains several proteolytic enzymes of digestion, such as trypsin and elastase, as well as enzymes of fat and carbohydrate digestion. Pancreatic exocrine secretion is controlled primarily by the hormones secretin and cholecystokinin, which are secreted by cells in the small intestinal mucosa.

386. The answer is C. *(Ganong, 15/e. pp 456–460.)* Secretion of acid by gastric parietal (oxyntic) epithelial cells is stimulated by histamine synthesized and released locally by enterochromaffin cells within the gastric mucosa. Histamine interacts with specific H_2 receptors on the gastric parietal cells and stimulates acid secretion by a cyclic AMP–dependent mechanism. Histamine is rapidly metabolized and inactivated, primarily by methylation. Cimetidine, as well as other H_2 receptor antagonists, blocks the histamine–H_2 receptor interaction without blocking other systemic effects of histamine. Vagal or parasympathetic stimulation enhances acid secretion via cholinergic stimulation of parietal cell secretion. Somatostatin is released from cells within the gastric mucosa and inhibits acid secretion by a paracrine mechanism.

387. The answer is C. *(Guyton, 8/e. pp 735, 742.)* The digestive tract normally contains about 150 to 200 mL of gas, most of which is in the colon, with approximately 50 mL in the stomach. Most of the gas in the stomach is derived from air swallowed during eating or in periods of anxiety. Gas is produced in the small intestine by interaction of gastric acid and bicarbonate in the intestinal and pancreatic secretions but does not accumulate because it is either reabsorbed or quickly passed into the colon. Gas within the colon is derived primarily from fermentation of undigested material by intestinal bacteria to produce CO_2, H_2, and methane. The amount of gas varies markedly from one person to another and is influenced by diet; e.g., ingestion of large amounts of beans, which contain undigestible carbohydrates in their hulls, will increase gas formation by intestinal bacteria. Diffusion of gas from the blood to the intestinal lumen is responsible for the N_2 present in intestinal gas and is influenced by the atmospheric pressure.

388. The answer is D. *(Berne, 2/e. pp 665–666, 696–697, 699.)* The distal stomach, which includes the antrum and the pyloric sphincter, is involved in the regulation of the gastric emptying of solids and in the regulation of secretion of acid. Antral peristaltic contractions are necessary for the adequate trituration of solids. The pyloric sphincter serves to limit the flow of solids out of the stomach until the particles are of a small enough size to be suspended in the liquid component of the meal. Removal of the antrum and the sphincter will increase the rate of gastric emptying because the resistance to flow of large particles will be removed. Secretion of acid will be decreased because of the loss of gastrin, which is normally secreted by the G cells of the antrum. Gastric compliance is a property of the proximal stomach.

389. The answer is B. *(Berne, 2/e. pp 730, 741.)* The terminal ileum contains specialized cells responsible for the absorption of primary and secondary bile salts by active transport. Bile salts are necessary for adequate digestion and absorption of fat. In the absence of the terminal ileum there will be an increase in the amounts of bile acids and fatty acids delivered to the colon. Fats and bile salts in the colon increase the water content of the feces by promoting the influx (secretion) of water into the lumen of the colon. Amino acids are absorbed in the jejunum. Iron is primarily absorbed in the duodenum.

390. The answer is E. *(Ganong, 15/e. p 474.)* Several vitamins—including vitamin K, several of the B complex, and folic acid—can be synthesized by intestinal bacteria. However, in humans, only folic acid so synthesized is absorbed by the host. Dietary intake of the other vitamins is necessary.

391. The answer is D. *(Ganong, 15/e. pp 456–457.)* The parietal cells of the gastric mucosa secrete acid in response to gastrin, acetylcholine, and histamine stimulation. Two different types of histamine receptors, H_1 and H_2, have been identified in the body. Gastric acid secretion is mediated by H_2 receptors, which are selectively inhibited by cimetidine, whereas antihistamines that are used clinically to treat the nasal and sinus congestion in allergic reactions act at H_1 receptors. Acid secretion is a process that requires energy for the active transport of H^+ and Cl^- and utilizes CO_2. The following net reaction illustrates the process, but does not describe the actual sequence of chemical reactions:

$$CO_2 + H_2O + NaCl \rightarrow HCl + NaHCO_3$$

Chief cells contain zymogen granules and secrete pepsinogens.

392. The answer is A. *(Ganong, 15/e. p 452.)* Gastric inhibitory peptide (GIP) is found in the K cells of the duodenal and jejunal mucosa. Its secretion is enhanced by oral administration of glucose or amino acids but not by intravenous infusion, indicating that GIP secretion is modulated by mucosal up-

take of nutrients. GIP secretion is inhibited by somatostatin, which is secreted locally in a paracrine fashion. The major physiologic actions of GIP
are (1) to decrease gastric motility and secretion and (2) to increase insulin
secretion.

393. The answer is A. *(Berne, 2/e. pp 728–730.)* The major route of absorption of sodium in the colon is electrogenic transport. Because of the "tight"
nature of the tight junctions that connect cells in the colon, a relatively large
potential difference exists between the musocal (negative) and serosal (positive) surfaces of the absorptive cells. This electrical difference favors the net
secretion of K^+ into the lumen. The amounts of absorption of Na^+ and secretion of K^+ can be affected by changes in levels of aldosterone. Secretion
of HCO_3^- occurs in exchange for absorption of Cl^-. No counterbalancing
cation exchange pumps are present in the colon. Bile acids in the colon would
hold water in the colon.

394. The answer is E. *(Berne, 2/e. pp 728–731.)* Fluid balance in the small
intestine and the colon is the summation of factors that favor absorption and
those that favor secretion. For example, bile salts and fatty acids in the colon
decrease absorption of water while at the same time they increase the flow of
water into the lumen. The net result is excess fluid loss. Similarly, a decrease
in the amount of water absorbed as a result of a decrease in neutral NaCl
absorption in the small intestine or as the result of the increased presence of
osmotic particles (nonabsorbable) in the small intestine may lead to diarrhea
if the increased volume presented to the colon exceeds the maximal daily
absorptive capacity of the colon (5 L per day).

395. The answer is E. *(Ganong, 15/e. pp 456–461.)* Gastric acid secretion is
regulated by both neural and local stimuli. The cephalic phase, which occurs
in response to smell or sight of food, is mediated by cholinergic fibers of the
vagus nerve that act either directly on parietal cells or stimulate gastrin release from G cells in the gastric mucosa. Gastrin is the major hormonal pro-
moter of gastric acid secretion and is released in response to the presence of
protein in the gastric lumen and in response to the hormone bombesin and to
cholinergic or beta-adrenergic stimulation. (Norepinephrine is primarily alpha-adrenergic.) Histamine is a potent stimulus for secretion of acid that is
produced locally in the stomach. Some effects of stimuli other than those of
histamine appear to be mediated in part by histamine since they are partially
blocked by cimetidine, a selective histamine H_2-receptor antagonist that has,
to a large extent, replaced surgery in the management of peptic ulcer disease.
Caffeine and alcohol stimulate acid secretion by direct action on the mucosa.

396. The answer is B. *(Ganong, 15/e. pp 437, 469–471. Guyton, 8/e. pp 729–731.)* The brush border on the luminal surface of the small intestine is formed by (1) microvilli on the surface of each epithelial cell and (2) an amorphous layer rich in neutral and amino sugars known as the glycocalyx, which forms a protective barrier. Within the brush border are numerous enzymes for hydrolysis of disaccharides, peptides, and nucleic acids, as well as specialized transport systems. The primary function of the brush border is to enhance absorption by increasing the surface area for transport. It has no role in movement of intestinal contents.

397. The answer is D. *(Berne, 2/e. pp 676–677.)* Migrating motor complexes (MMCs) are periods of intense electrical and contractile activity that occur at intervals in the interdigestive period. In humans, MMCs occur every 75 to 90 min and appear to involve both a neural input via the intrinsic nervous system and a hormonal input (motilin). The plasma level of motilin rises in concert with the generation of the MMC. Although they were originally described as occurring only in the small intestine, it is now well known that MMCs are present in the stomach and perhaps in the esophagus.

398. The answer is C. *(Berne, 2/e. pp 701–707.)* Pancreatic secretion is under both neural and hormonal control. Neurol control is by way of the vagus nerve and involves acetylcholine-mediated increases in enzymatic secretion. Hormonal stimulation of the pancreas is due to secretin, which increases output of water and bicarbonate, and cholecystokinin, which increases enzymatic output. Histamine plays a role in the regulation of secretion of gastric acid.

399. The answer is D. *(Ganong, 15/e. p 468. Guyton, 8/e. p 722.)* Contraction of the gallbladder and relaxation of the sphincter of Oddi at the junction of the common bile duct and duodenum are necessary for delivery of bile into the duodenum. These muscular actions are under both hormonal and neural control. Cholecystokinin is a peptide secreted by the duodenal mucosa in response to entry of food, especially fatty acids and amino acids. The hormone acts to promote gallbladder contraction and probably to relax the sphincter of Oddi; it also elicits secretion of enzyme-rich pancreatic juice. Vagal stimulation, which is cholinergically mediated and blocked by atropine, also promotes gallbladder contraction.

400. The answer is E. *(Ganong, 15/e. p 460. Guyton, 8/e. pp 702–703.)* The enterogastric reflex inhibits the activity of the pyloric pump and slows gastric emptying. It is mediated primarily by afferent fibers of the vagus nerve that transmit impulses to nuclei in the brainstem. Some direct transmission of impulses via the myenteric plexus also occurs. The reflex is elicited by irritation of the small bowel, increased duodenal pressure, excessive protein catabolites in the duodenum, or the presence of acid chyme in that part of the small intestine (pancreatic juice is alkaline). It acts to slow gastric emptying, thus permitting sufficient time for digestion and absorption of duodenal contents.

401. The answer is C. *(Berne, 2/e. pp 669–670.)* Acidification of the small intestine causes release of the hormone secretin. Secretin is the primary stimulus for pancreatic secretion of water and bicarbonate. In addition secretin may serve as an enterogastrone, i.e., a hormone involved in the inhibitory feedback regulation of gastric function. Cholecystokinin (CCK) is the hormone responsible for contraction of the gallbladder and relaxation of the sphincter of Oddi.

402. The answer is E. *(Berne, 2/e. pp 708–715.)* The conversion of cholesterol to primary bile acids takes place in the liver. Secondary bile acids are formed in the small intestine as a consequence of bacterial alteration of the primary bile acids. In order for both the primary and the secondary bile acids to be effective in promoting the digestion and absorption of fats, it is necessary that they form aggregates called *micelles*. Conjugation of the bile salts with glycine or taurine greatly enhances the probability of formation of micelles. Secretin is responsible for stimulation of the bile acid–independent fraction of bile. The presence of any osmotically active particles in the colon holds water in the stool and decreases water absorption.

403. The answer is C. *(Ganong, 15/e. pp 451–452, 456–462. Guyton, 8/e. pp 713–715, 718–719.)* Mucus and intrinsic factor are both secreted by the gastric mucosa, i.e., the mucosa of the stomach. Mucus protects the epithelium and provides a lubricant for food transport. Intrinsic factor, secreted by the parietal cells, is important for the absorption of cyanocobalamin (vitamin B_{12}) by the distal ileum. Cholecystokinin, which is secreted by the duodenum, enhances release of enzyme-rich pancreatic juice and contraction and emptying of the gallbladder. Secretin is also secreted by the duodenum and enhances secretion of the watery, alkaline portion of pancreatic juice. Trypsinogen is a constituent of the pancreatic juice and is converted to trypsin by enteropeptidase (enterokinase) in the small intestine.

404. The answer is E. *(Ganong, 15/e. p 455.)* There is no discrete muscular band at the gastroesophageal junction that forms an anatomic lower esophageal sphincter (LES). Intraluminal pressure measurements have demonstrated a segment 4 to 6 cm in length beginning about 2 cm above the diaphragm in which intraluminal pressure is increased by an increase in muscle tone so that this segment functions as a physiologic sphincter. Tonic activity of this sphincter between meals prevents reflux of acidic gastric contents into the esophagus, whose squamous mucosa lacks a protective mucous coating. During swallowing, this segment relaxes to permit passage of the swallowed material into the stomach. The esophagus is innervated by both sympathetic and parasympathetic divisions of the autonomic system. In achalasia, the tension in the lower esophageal sphincter is increased by pathologic changes in the vagal fibers, so that food accumulates in the esophagus, which becomes markedly dilated. During pregnancy, the resting tension in the lower esophageal sphincter is decreased. This is a contributing factor in the increase in acid reflux during pregnancy.

405. The answer is C. *(Berne, 2/e. pp 696–700.)* Paracrine secretions are locally released chemicals that act to alter the biologic activity of the surrounding cells. Histamine and somatostatin are paracrine secretions that are involved in the regulation of secretion of acid by the stomach. Histamine is a stimulus for secretion of acid. Its activity is necessary for the full expression of secretion of gastric acid. Somatostatin acts to locally regulate secretion of acid by decreasing the secretory capacity of the parietal cell and by decreasing the amount of gastrin released from antral G cells. Gastrin, cholecystokinin, and secretin are hormones that act on the gastrointestinal system after being released into the circulation.

406. The answer is D. *(Ganong, 15/e. pp 438, 441.)* Protein digestion begins with the action of pepsins in the stomach. Because pepsins require a pH of 1.6 to 3.2, they are rendered inactive when they reach the more alkaline environment of the duodenum. Trypsin, chymotrypsin, elastase, and carboxypeptidase all are proteolytic enzymes that are active in the intestine.

407. The answer is E. *(Ganong, 15/e. pp 465–467.)* Cholic, chenodeoxycholic, deoxycholic, and lithocholic acids all have been isolated from human bile. The sodium and potassium salts of these acids (bile salts) are important in emulsification and the formation of micelles for fat absorption. They also activate intestinal lipases and stimulate glycerol synthesis and reesterification of fatty acids.

408. The answer is D. *(Berne, 2/e. pp 661–664.)* The term *primary esophageal peristalsis* denotes that swallowing has been elicited as a consequence of activation of the "swallowing centers" in the medulla. The event involves not only esophageal peristalsis and relaxation of the lower esophageal sphincter (LES), but also the transit of food through the pharyngeal region. It is initiated via the vagus nerve. Secondary esophageal peristalsis is a localized esophageal response to irritation or distention that results in a peristaltic contraction and relaxation of the LES. Both primary and secondary esophageal peristalses involve the intrinsic nervous system.

409. The answer is C. *(Ganong, 15/e. p 446.)* Absorption of the fat-soluble vitamins (A, D, E, and K) is diminished if there is a lack of bile or pancreatic lipase. Lipase is required to produce monoglycerides that, in combination with bile salts, make it possible to bring the fat-soluble vitamins close to the mucosal cell surface for absorption. With the exception of vitamin B_{12}, which is absorbed bound to intrinsic factor in the ileum, vitamins are absorbed chiefly in the upper small intestine.

410. The answer is E. *(Guyton, 8/e. pp 46–49, 733.)* The following four statements about intestinal absorption of monosaccharides support the idea that their transport is an active process: transport can be blocked by metabolic inhibitors; transport is selective for different sugars; a maximum rate of transport exists for individual monosaccharides; and competition exists among sugars for the carrier mechanism. These principles also apply to the active transport of monosaccharides through the renal tubular membranes. As a result, it is assumed that the same mechanism is involved in both sites.

Neurophysiology

DIRECTIONS: Each question below contains five suggested responses. Select the **one best** response to each question.

411. The primary function of the bones of the middle ear in human hearing is to

(A) amplify the sound stimulus
(B) filter high-frequency sounds from the sound stimulus
(C) enable the direction of a sound stimulus to be detected
(D) enhance the ability to distinguish different sound frequencies
(E) protect the ear from damage

412. Which one of the following will most likely cause body temperature to remain above normal?

(A) A decrease in the amount of blood flowing to the skin
(B) An increase in the intensity of exercise
(C) An increase in the set point of the thermoregulatory system
(D) An increase in production of thyroxine
(E) A decrease in the amount of evaporative water loss

413. An aphasia is most likely to be associated with a lesion of

(A) the hippocampus
(B) Broca's area
(C) the parietal lobe
(D) the limbic system
(E) the reticular activating system

414. All the following neurotransmitters are inactivated when diffused out of the cleft or pumped into the presynaptic nerve ending EXCEPT

(A) serotonin
(B) glycine
(C) norepinephrine
(D) dopamine
(E) acetylcholine

415. Which of the following structures is most responsible for the observation that not all frequencies of sound have the same threshold?

(A) Outer ear
(B) Middle ear
(C) Inner ear
(D) Tectorial membrane
(E) Basilar membrane

416. In the accompanying graph, brief repetitive stimulation of a presynaptic neuron is followed by a prolonged interval in which a much lower voltage is required to elicit a postsynaptic response. This phenomenon, termed *posttetanic potentiation,* is due to

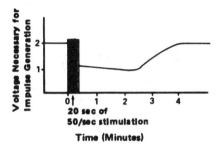

Time (Minutes)

(A) enhanced synthesis of neurotransmitter
(B) increased axoplasmic transport in the presynaptic cell
(C) accumulation of calcium in the presynaptic terminal
(D) altered affinity of the postsynaptic receptor for neurotransmitter
(E) decreased catabolism of neurotransmitter in the junctional space

417. The hypothalamus is LEAST involved in the regulation of

(A) intake of water
(B) temperature
(C) osmolarity of urine
(D) respiration
(E) emotional behavior

418. Presynaptic inhibition in the central nervous system affects the sensitivity of motor neurons by inducing all the following changes EXCEPT

(A) an elevation of the resting potential of the excitatory nerve endings
(B) an increase in the excitability of the excitatory nerve endings
(C) a partial depolarization of the excitatory nerve endings
(D) a reduction in excitatory nerve membrane potential
(E) a decrease in the amount of mediator liberated at the synapse

419. The most important role of the gamma motoneurons is to

(A) stimulate skeletal muscle fibers to contract
(B) maintain Ia afferent activity during contraction of muscle
(C) generate activity in Ib afferent fibers
(D) detect the length of resting skeletal muscle
(E) prevent muscles from producing too much force

420. The myotatic stretch reflex uses the smallest number of neurons of any cord reflex. Stretch of a muscle spindle causes all the following events EXCEPT

(A) excitation of receptors
(B) excitation of motor nerves
(C) transmission of impulses to anterior motor neurons
(D) a static as well as dynamic reflex
(E) relaxation of muscle

421. The accompanying figure is a schematic diagram of a myoneural junction of a skeletal muscle. Substance 1 is the neurotransmitter released by the nerve that stimulates the muscle cell membrane to depolarize. With stimulation of the muscle cell membrane, ion 2 rushes intracellularly and ion 3 rushes extracellularly. Substances 1, 2, and 3 are, respectively,

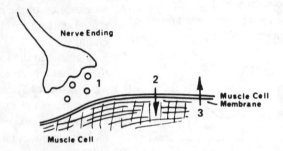

(A) acetylcholine, chloride, sodium
(B) acetylcholine, sodium, potassium
(C) acetylcholine, potassium, sodium
(D) norepinephrine, sodium, chloride
(E) norepinephrine, sodium, potassium

---

422. Which of the following determines whether release of neurotransmitter at synaptic junctions results in an excitatory or inhibitory effect on postsynaptic neurons?

(A) The chemical structure of the neurotransmitter
(B) The properties of the postsynaptic receptor
(C) The rate of reuptake of neurotransmitter by the presynaptic cell
(D) The amount of calcium released from presynaptic axons
(E) The velocity of axoplasmic transport in the presynaptic neuron

423. The middle cerebellar peduncle contains afferent fibers conveyed in which of the following tracts?

(A) Dorsal spinocerebellar
(B) Ventral spinocerebellar
(C) Tectocerebellar
(D) Pontocerebellar
(E) Vestibulocerebellar

424. The precentral gyrus and corticospinal tract are essential for

(A) vision
(B) olfaction
(C) auditory identification
(D) kinesthesia
(E) voluntary movement

425. A patient who presents with an intention tremor, scanning speech, "past-pointing," and a "drunken" gait might be expected to have a lesion involving the

(A) cerebellum
(B) medulla
(C) cortical motor strip
(D) basal ganglia
(E) eighth cranial nerve

426. Which of the following statements about the hair cells of the cochlea is true?

(A) They protect the lower airways from large particulate matter
(B) They support the basilar membrane
(C) They are connected by neural pathways to the lateral geniculate body
(D) They are contained in the macula
(E) They are vestigial organs without function

427. One of the reactions in the retinal rods directly caused by absorption of light energy is

(A) dissociation of scotopsin and metarhodopsin
(B) decomposition of scotopsin
(C) transformation of *cis* retinene to *trans* retinene
(D) transformation of metarhodopsin to lumirhodopsin
(E) transformation of vitamin A to retinene

428. Mydriasis, or pupillary dilatation, involves all the following EXCEPT

(A) contraction of the radial fibers of the iris
(B) relaxation of the sphincter muscles of the iris
(C) stimulation of the Edinger-Westphal nucleus
(D) sympathetic nerve discharge
(E) impulse transmission by the superior cervical ganglion

429. All the following statements about the eye are true EXCEPT that the

(A) focal point of a hyperopic eye is behind the retina
(B) focal point of a myopic eye is in front of the retina
(C) focal point of an emmetropic eye is on the retina
(D) vision in a myopic eye can be corrected by use of a biconvex lens
(E) ciliary muscle is relaxed in an emmetropic eye focusing on an object 40 feet away

430. The Renshaw cell functions by repetitively and rapidly transmitting an impulse to a motor neuron and causing it to become hyperpolarized. This results in

(A) stimulation of the motor neuron
(B) inhibition of the motor neuron
(C) transmission of the impulse to other motor neurons
(D) "reverse" transmission of the impulse down a sensory neuron
(E) none of the above

431. Which of the following statements about the cerebrospinal fluid (CSF) is true?

(A) It is absorbed by the choroid plexus
(B) Its absorption is independent of CSF pressure
(C) It circulates in the epidural space
(D) It has a lower glucose concentration than plasma
(E) It has a higher protein concentration than plasma

432. When a person slowly rotates toward the right,

(A) the stereocilia on the hair cells in the right horizontal semicircular canal bend away from the kinocilium
(B) both the left and right eyes deviate toward the left
(C) the hair cells in the left horizontal semicircular canal become depolarized
(D) the visual image on the retina becomes unfocused
(E) the endolymph in the left and right horizontal semicircular canals moves in opposite directions

433. Correct statements regarding rapid eye movement (REM) sleep include which of the following?

(A) It is the first state of sleep entered when a person falls asleep
(B) It is accompanied by loss of skeletal muscle tone
(C) It is characterized by a slow but steady heart rate
(D) It occurs more often in adults than in children
(E) It lasts longer than periods of slow-wave sleep

434. When emmetropic persons become presbyopic, their

(A) visual acuity increases
(B) near point increases
(C) far point decreases
(D) total refractive power increases
(E) ability to see distant objects decreases

435. When light strikes the eye, which of the following will increase?

(A) The sodium conductance of the photoreceptors
(B) The amount of transmitter released from the photoreceptors
(C) The concentration of rhodopsin in the photoreceptors
(D) The membrane potential of the photoreceptors
(E) The concentration of cyclic guanosine monophosphate (cGMP)

436. Spasticity can be caused by sectioning

(A) the corticospinal fibers
(B) the vestibulospinal fibers
(C) the Ia afferent fibers
(D) the corticoreticular fibers
(E) the reticulospinal fibers

437. Light shining on the retina will result in which of the following events?

(A) Activation of the nuclei of rod photoreceptors
(B) Conversion of guanosine triphosphate (GTP) to cyclic guanosine monophosphate (cGMP)
(C) Generation of *cis*-retinal from rhodopsin
(D) Depolarization of cone photoreceptors
(E) Activation of a phosphodiesterase enzyme

438. The cerebellum is important in controlling

(A) muscular coordination
(B) stereognosis
(C) muscle strength
(D) stretch reflexes
(E) posture

439. The alpha rhythm appearing on an electroencephalogram has which of the following characteristics?

(A) It produces 20 to 30 waves per second
(B) It disappears when a patient's eyes open
(C) It is replaced by slower, larger waves during REM sleep
(D) It represents activity that is most pronounced in the frontal region of the brain
(E) It is associated with deep sleep

440. Tapping the patella tendon elicits a reflex contraction of the quadriceps muscle. During the contraction of the quadriceps muscle,

(A) the Ib afferents from the Golgi tendon organ increase their rate of firing
(B) the Ia afferents from the muscle spindle increase their rate of firing
(C) the alpha motoneurons innervating the muscle spindles decrease their rate of firing
(D) the gamma motoneurons innervating the muscle spindles increase their rate of firing
(E) the alpha motoneurons to the antagonistic muscles increase their rate of firing

441. Visual accommodation involves which of the following mechanisms?

(A) Release of norepinephrine by sympathetic nerve fibers
(B) A decrease in the thickness of the lens
(C) Relaxation of the ciliary muscle
(D) Stretch of the lens suspensory ligaments
(E) A decrease in the focal length of the eye

442. The vestibular apparatus is characterized by all the following EXCEPT

(A) the ability to detect linear acceleration via the macula
(B) the ability to detect angular acceleration via the cristae ampullaris
(C) the presence of endolymph in the membranous semicircular canals
(D) an afferent neural connection with the central nervous system via cranial nerve VIII
(E) the ability to produce a conscious sensation

443. Beta receptors activate G proteins that activate

(A) adenyl cyclase
(B) protein kinase A
(C) protein kinase C
(D) calmodulin
(E) phospholipase C

444. Norepinephrine will cause contraction of the smooth muscle in the

(A) bronchioles
(B) pupils
(C) intestine
(D) arterioles
(E) ciliary body

DIRECTIONS: Each group of questions below consists of four lettered headings followed by a set of numbered items. For each numbered item select

A	if the item is associated with	(A) **only**
B	if the item is associated with	(B) **only**
C	if the item is associated with	**both** (A) and (B)
D	if the item is associated with	**neither** (A) nor (B)

Each lettered heading may be used **once, more than once, or not at all.**

Questions 445–449

  (A) Sympathetic
  (B) Parasympathetic
  (C) Both
  (D) Neither

445. Postganglionic neurons located in the effector organs

446. Preganglionic fibers that secrete acetylcholine at their synaptic terminals

447. Postganglionic fibers that may be either cholinergic or adrenergic

448. Preganglionic neurons localized in cervical and sacral regions

449. Postganglionic neurons located in discrete ganglia

Questions 450–454

  (A) Golgi tendon organ
  (B) Muscle spindle
  (C) Both
  (D) Neither

450. Will be hyperactive in spasticity

451. Will increase its activity upon gamma motoneuron discharge

452. Will increase its activity during a muscle contraction

453. Will indicate the amount of tension generated by a muscle

454. Will cause a reflex relaxation of the muscle in which it is located

DIRECTIONS: Each group of questions below consists of lettered headings followed by a set of numbered items. For each numbered item select the **one** lettered heading with which it is **most** closely associated. Each lettered heading may be used **once, more than once, or not at all.**

Questions 455–458

For each abnormality listed below, select the visual field defect (black area) that it is most likely to produce. Answer E if none of the options apply.

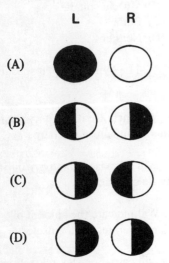

Questions 459–460

Match each description with one of the points on the action potential diagrammed below.

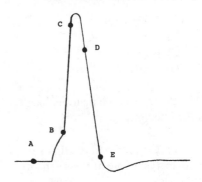

459. The point at which the driving force for potassium is the greatest

460. The point at which sodium conductance is greatest

455. Interruption of left optic nerve

456. Interruption of optic chiasma

457. Interruption of left optic tract

458. Enlargement of pituitary gland

Neurophysiology
Answers

411. The answer is A. *(Berne, 2/e. pp 162–164.)* When sound waves pass from air to water, most of the energy contained in the sound stimulus is lost. Because the auditory receptors within the inner ear are bathed in liquid, most of the energy in the sound stimulus potentially could be lost as the sound travels from air to water. The bones of the middle ear significantly reduce the amount of loss by amplifying the sound stimulus. Most of the amplification results from the much larger surface area of the tympanic membrane compared with that of the oval window (or from the larger area of the malleus compared with that of the stapes). The reduction in area focuses the sound stimulus onto a smaller area, thus increasing the sound pressure. Audiologists refer to this amplification phenomenon as *impedance matching*.

412. The answer is C. *(Ganong, 15/e. pp 234–235, 302–303, 587.)* When a person is exposed to a cold environment, the thermoregulatory system responds by activating a number of heat-conserving or heat-producing mechanisms. These include a decrease in blood supply to the skin, a decrease in sweating, an increase in shivering (or exercise), and an increase in metabolic activity brought about by an increase in shivering, exercise, or production of thyroxine. Although all of these mechanisms may increase body temperature above normal, they usually are evoked to bring body temperature back to normal. However, if the set point is increased (e.g., by a fever), the activity of the heat-conserving mechanisms will increase and those mechanisms that bring about a loss of heat will decrease, which will cause a rise in temperature.

413. The answer is B. *(Berne, 2/e. pp 264–266.)* Aphasia is a language disorder in which a person is unable to properly express or understand certain aspects of written or spoken language. It is caused by lesions to the language centers of the brain, which, for the majority of persons, are located within the left hemisphere in the portions of the temporal and frontal lobes known as Wernicke's and Broca's areas, respectively. Language disorders caused by memory loss, which could be the result of a hippocampal lesion, are not classified as aphasias.

414. The answer is E. *(Ganong, 15/e. pp 89–94, 98.)* The action of acetylcholine (ACh) is terminated by acetylcholinesterase (AChE), which hydrolyzes ACh to acetate and choline. The choline is pumped into the nerve terminal and used in the resynthesis of new ACh. All other transmitters are inactivated by reuptake into the nerve terminal. A variety of drugs act by preventing reuptake of the neurotransmitter into the nerve terminal or, in the case of ACh, by blocking the action of AChE.

415. The answer is B. *(Ganong, 15/e. pp 165–166.)* In order for sounds to be detected by the ear, they must pass from the air to the fluid medium of the inner ear. For this to occur, the sound pressure must be amplified (or an impedance match between air and fluid must be created). The large difference in surface area between the tympanic membrane and oval window of the middle ear provides for this amplification (or impedance matching). However, not all frequencies are equally amplified; certain frequencies, those between 500 and 5000 Hz, are heard at much lower sound pressures than are lower or higher frequencies.

416. The answer is C. *(Ganong, 15/e. p 101.)* Synaptic transmission involves release of neurotransmitter synthesized in the presynaptic terminal and interaction of this neurotransmitter with a specific receptor in the postsynaptic cell membrane. Stimulation of the presynaptic cell also results in an influx of calcium into the presynaptic terminal from the extracellular fluid. This influx of calcium is required for the release of neurotransmitter by exocytosis. Brief repetitive stimulation results in accumulation of calcium within the presynaptic cell, so that subsequent stimulation with a lower voltage, which results in a correspondingly lower influx of calcium, is sufficient to permit efficient excitation-secretion coupling. This enhancement persists until calcium stores are depleted. It is not dependent on catabolism or synthesis of neurotransmitter and is independent of transport of axoplasmic protein and the postsynaptic receptor. The physiologic significance of this phenomenon is unclear, but posttetanic potentiation may function in short-term storage of information.

417. The answer is D. *(Berne, 2/e. pp 288–296.)* The hypothalamus contains osmoreceptors responsible for detecting increases in extracellular osmolarity. These osmoreceptors produce the sensation of thirst, increase drinking, and cause the release of antidiuretic hormone (ADH). Thermoreceptors in the anterior hypothalamus measure core temperature. Other hypothalamic neurons are involved in the initiation and coordination of heat-conserving and heat-losing mechanisms. The hypothalamus also serves as a component of the limbic system, which is responsible, in part, for mediating emotional behavior. Respiration is controlled by respiratory centers of the brainstem.

418. The answer is A. *(Ganong, 15/e. p 83.)* Presynaptic inhibition is caused by interneurons that interact with axons of excitatory neurons and secrete a transmitter that induces a partial depolarization of the excitatory neuron. The membrane potential of the excitatory nerve ending is reduced; thus it is more easily excited because less stimulation is required to achieve the threshold for an action potential. However, because the resting potential is lower, the voltage of the action potential is reduced by the same amount. Inasmuch as the amount of mediator released at the synapse is related to the magnitude of the action potential, less transmitter is released and there is less postsynaptic cell excitation.

419. The answer is B. *(Berne, 2/e. pp 200–206.)* The gamma motoneurons innervate the intrafusal fibers of the muscle spindles. When a skeletal muscle contracts, the intrafusal muscle fiber becomes slack and the Ia afferents stop firing. By stimulating the intrafusal muscle fibers during a contraction, the gamma motoneurons prevent the intrafusal muscle fibers from becoming slack and thus maintain Ia firing during the contraction.

420. The answer is E. *(Ganong, 15/e. pp 115–119.)* The myotatic—or stretch—reflex, which is a spinal cord reflex that prevents further stretch of muscle by stimulating contraction of muscle fiber, is important in preventing oscillation and jerking movements. It is mediated by a specialized muscle fiber, the muscle spindle, which, when stretched, transmits impulses via the dorsal root to motor neurons in the anterior horn of the spinal cord. The reflex is normally subject to both facilitation and inhibition by higher centers.

421. The answer is B. *(Ganong, 15/e. pp 88–89, 102–103.)* At rest, the difference in electrical potential across the membrane of the muscle cell (resting potential) is −90 millivolts. The nerve releases acetylcholine, which changes the ionic permeability of the muscle plasma membrane. Owing to the differences in concentration of sodium ions (high outside) and potassium ions (high inside) across the membrane, the increased permeability to ions gives rise to a sudden influx of sodium and efflux of potassium ions through the plasma membrane. This results in depolarization of the muscle membrane.

422. The answer is B. *(Berne, 2/e. pp 60–65.)* Release of neurotransmitter from presynaptic cells is accompanied by an influx of calcium from the extracellular fluid. The neurotransmitter then interacts with receptors on the plasma membrane of the postsynaptic cell. It is the specificity of these receptors that determines whether the net effect is inhibitory or excitatory. A specific transmitter may have either effect depending on the site of action. Thus, acetylcholine is excitatory at the neuromuscular junction but is inhibitory when released by the vagus nerve at cardiac muscle junctions.

423. The answer is D. *(Berne, 2/e. pp 227–232.)* The middle cerebellar peduncle contains afferent fibers conveyed in the pontocerebellar tract, which carries impulses from the motor area as well as other parts of the cerebellar cortex except the flocculonodular lobe. The dorsal spinocerebellar and vestibulocerebellar afferent tracts enter the cerebellum via the inferior peduncle. The ventral spinocerebellar and tectocerebellar tracts enter via the superior cerebellar peduncle.

424. The answer is E. *(Berne, 2/e. pp 249–252.)* The precentral gyrus is the motor area of the cortex and the corticospinal tract is the pyramidal tract proper. These two structures are essential for voluntary movement. A supplementary motor area, whose function is still unknown, exists on the medial side of the hemisphere.

425. The answer is A. *(Ganong, 15/e. pp 200–201, 205–206.)* Ataxia, scanning speech, dysmetria, and an intention tremor all are classic findings in a patient with a lesion involving the cerebellum. Affected persons also exhibit adiadochokinesia, which is a loss of ability to accomplish a swift succession of oscillatory movements, such as external and internal rotation of the foot. These symptoms all result from destruction of the normal feedback mechanisms that are coordinated in the cerebellum.

426. The answer is D. *(Ganong, 15/e. pp 159–163.)* The cochlear hair cells are the functioning auditory receptors. Neural pathways from the hair cells pass to the inferior colliculi and the medial geniculate body before synapsing in the auditory cortex. The hair cells are contained in the macula (otolithic organ) and are overlaid by the otolithic membrane.

427. The answer is C. *(Ganong, 15/e. pp 139–140, 144–147.)* The light-sensitive chemical in the retinal rods is called *rhodopsin*. It is a combination of retinene (in the *cis* configuration) and scotopsin. Light immediately changes the *cis* structure of retinene to the *trans* structure. Other reactions follow because the physical structure of the *trans* retinene no longer combines in a stable fashion with scotopsin. Rhodopsin's decomposition upon exposure to light excites the nerve fibers in the eye.

428. The answer is C. *(West, 12/e. pp 972, 975–976.)* Sympathetic nerves from the superior cervical ganglion innervate the radial fibers of the iris, and their excitation induces pupillary dilatation. Constriction of the pupil in response to light is mediated via afferent fibers to the pretectal area of the pons, from which efferent fibers pass to the nucleus of Edinger-Westphal. From that point, parasympathetic cholinergic fibers pass via the ciliary ganglion to the ciliary muscles and sphincter of the iris. When dilatation of the pupil occurs, the nucleus of Edinger-Westphal is inhibited.

429. The answer is D. *(Ganong, 15/e. pp 143–144.)* Biconcave (not biconvex) lenses cause light rays to diverge and, when placed in front of a myopic (nearsighted) eye, will move the focal point back until it reaches the retina, which is required to correct nearsightedness. In hyperopia (farsightedness), the eyeball is decreased in anteroposterior diameter, resulting in a focal point that lies *behind* the retina; in myopia, this diameter is increased, causing the focal point to lie in *front* of the retina. Emmetropia refers to an optically normal eye. In astigmatism, another common refractive error, the curvature of the cornea is nonspherical.

430. The answer is B. *(Ganong, 15/e. pp 81–82. West, 12/e. pp 58–59.)* Renshaw cells are interneurons that are activated by a branch of a motor neuron and release inhibitory neurotransmitters. The inhibitory transmitter hyperpolarizes the motor neuron and renders it less susceptible to depolarization. Such negative feedback inhibition by neurons also occurs in the cerebral cortex and limbic system. Renshaw cells are often associated with motor neurons of the spinal cord.

431. The answer is D. *(Ganong, 15/e. pp 563–565.)* Cerebrospinal fluid (CSF), which is in osmotic equilibrium with the extracellular fluid of the brain and spinal cord, is formed primarily in the choroid plexus by an active secretory process. It circulates through the subarachnoid space between the dura mater and pia mater and is absorbed into the circulation by the arachnoid villi. The epidural space, which lies outside the dura mater, may be used clinically for instillation of anesthetics. CSF protein and glucose concentrations are much lower than those of plasma. Changes in those concentrations in the CSF are helpful in detecting pathologic processes, e.g., tumor or infection, in which the blood-brain barrier is disrupted.

432. The answer is B. *(Berne, 2/e. pp 180–186.)* When the head rotates in one direction, the hair cells mounted on the cristae rotate along with the head. However, the flow of endolymph is delayed and as a result the cupula is moved in a direction opposite to the movement of the head. When the head moves to the right, the cupula moves toward the left; this bends the stereocilia on the hair cells in the right horizontal canal toward the kinocilium and bends the stereocilia on the hair cells in the left horizontal canal toward the kinocilium. As a result the hair cells in the right horizontal canal depolarize and those in the left horizontal canal hyperpolarize. The depolarization of the hair cells in the right horizontal canal stimulates the right vestibular nerve, which in turn causes the eyes to deviate toward the left. The movement of the eyes toward the left as the head deviates toward the right keeps the image on the retina in focus.

433. The answer is B. *(Berne, 2/e. pp 266–268.)* In a normal sleep cycle, a person passes through the four stages of slow-wave sleep before entering REM sleep. In narcolepsy, a person may pass directly from the waking state to REM sleep. REM sleep is characterized by irregular heart beats and respiration and by periods of atonia (loss of muscle tone). It is also the state of sleep in which dreaming occurs.

434. The answer is B. *(Ganong, 15/e. pp 142–144.)* In presbyopia, the ability of the lens to accommodate for near vision decreases. Thus the total refractive power of the eye decreases and the ability of the eye to form a focused image of objects placed close to it decreases. The near point is the closest point to which an object can be brought and still remain in focus. This increases when the accommodative power of the eye is decreased. There is no effect on the far point or visual acuity; these remain normal.

435. The answer is D. *(Ganong, 15/e. pp 144–146.)* When light strikes the eye and is absorbed by rhodopsin, a photoisomerization of 11-*cis* retinal to all-*trans* retinal occurs. As a consequence of this photoisomerization, rhodopsin is activated. The rhodopsin then activates transducin, which in turn activates a phosphodiesterase, which hydrolyzes cGMP. When cGMP concentrations within the rods or cones decrease, sodium channels close, sodium conductance decreases, and the cell hyperpolarizes. Hyperpolarization of the cell causes a decrease in the release of neurotransmitter. Eventually the all-*trans* retinal dissociates from opsin and reduces the concentration of rhodopsin in the cell.

436. The answer is D. *(Berne, 2/e. pp 225–226.)* Spasticity results from overactivity of the alpha motoneurons innervating the skeletal musculature. Under normal circumstances, these alpha motoneurons are tonically stimulated by reticulospinal and vestibulospinal fibers originating in the brainstem.

These brainstem fibers are normally inhibited by fibers originating in the cortex. Cutting the cortical fibers releases the brainstem fibers from inhibition and results in spasticity. Cutting the fibers from the reticular formation or vestibular nuclei or the Ia afferents will reduce the spasticity.

437. The answer is E. *(Berne, 2/e. pp 16–21. Ganong, 15/e. pp 144–146.)* The retina contains two types of photoreceptors: rods, which function in gray level discrimination, and cones, which are important in light and color vision. These receptor cells derive their names from their shapes, and their shapes are determined by their complex plasma membrane, which comprises hundreds to thousands of disk-shaped structures containing photopigments. When light shines on the retina, it interacts with these disks and causes *cis-trans* isomerization of retinal, the prosthetic group associated with the photoreceptor proteins. This isomerization is associated with hydrolysis of cGMP by a light-sensitive cGMP phosphodiesterase and with hyperpolarization of the plasma membrane caused by a decrease in sodium conductance across the membrane. The nucleus of the photoreceptor cell has no known role in the response to light.

438. The answer is A. *(Ganong, 15/e. pp 202–206.)* The primary function of the cerebellum is to coordinate muscular activity throughout the body. It does so without directly controlling muscular contraction but by receiving input from the periphery and cerebral motor areas and comparing the actual position of each part of the body with the position intended by motor centers. Pain sensation is mediated by afferent fibers that interact primarily with the thalamus and parietal cortex. Stereognosis, the recognition of objects by touch without vision, is mediated by the cortex.

439. The answer is B. *(Ganong, 15/e. pp 180–182.)* In a totally relaxed adult with eyes closed, the major component of the electroencephalogram (EEG) will be a regular pattern of 8 to 12 waves per second, called the *alpha rhythm*. The alpha rhythm disappears when the eyes are opened. It is most prominent in the parietooccipital region. In deep sleep, the alpha rhythm is replaced by larger, slower waves called *delta waves*. In REM sleep, the EEG will show fast, irregular activity.

440. The answer is A. *(Berne, 2/e. pp 200–208.)* Stretching the patella tendon stretches the muscle spindles within the quadriceps muscle and causes an increase in Ia afferent activity. The increase in Ia afferent activity causes an increase in alpha motoneuron activity, which results in contraction of the quadriceps muscle. When the muscle contracts, the muscle spindles are unloaded and the Ia afferent activity is reduced. However, the Ib activity is increased during contraction because of the tension placed on the Golgi tendon organs.

441. The answer is E. *(Ganong, 15/e. pp 140–143.)* When an object is brought nearer to the eye, it is kept in focus by increasing the refractive power of the eye. Increasing the refractive power of the eye causes a decrease in the focal length. Refractive power is increased by the accommodation reflex, which is initiated by parasympathetic fibers that contract the ciliary muscle. This allows the suspensory ligaments to retract, which in turn permits the lens to thicken and increase its curvature. The increase in curvature causes the increase in the refractive power of the eye.

442. The answer is E. *(Ganong, 15/e. pp 169–170.)* In the vestibular apparatus the macula is located in the utricle and the cristae ampullaris are located in the ampullae of the semicircular canals. The macula and the cristae ampullaris have similar structures containing hair cells that are stimulated by otoconia. Maculae, being sensitive to changes in gravitational pull, are able to detect *linear* acceleration; ampullar structures, being sensitive to changes in the flow of endolymph in the semicircular canals, are able to detect *angular* acceleration. Sensory nerve fibers are transmitted via cranial nerve VIII to the vestibular nuclei. Although the vestibular apparatus produces a feeling of up and down and of movement, no particular conscious sensation results from vestibular nerve activity.

443. The answer is A. *(Ganong, 15/e. pp 33–39.)* Beta-receptor activated G proteins activate adenyl cyclase, which catalyzes the production of cAMP from ATP. The cAMP then activates protein kinase A, which produces its physiologic effects by phosphorylating a variety of proteins. Phospholipase C is activated by a G protein, which is activated by muscarinic and alpha$_1$-adrenergic receptors. Phospholipase C hydrolyzes PIP$_2$ and thus produces IP$_3$ and DAG. Protein kinase C is in turn activated by DAG.

444. The answer is D. *(Ganong, 15/e. pp 210–212.)* The catecholamines norepinephrine and epinephrine will activate both alpha- and beta-adrenergic receptors. When the alpha$_1$-adrenergic receptors are stimulated they activate a G protein, which in turn activates phospholipase C that hydrolyzes PIP$_2$ and produces IP$_3$ and DAG. The IP$_3$ causes the release of Ca^{2+} from the sarcoplasmic reticulum, which in turn increases muscle contraction. Alpha$_1$-adrenergic receptors predominate on arteriolar smooth muscle, so these muscles contract when stimulated with norepinephrine. The bronchiolar, pupillary, and ciliary smooth muscles all contain beta receptors, which cause smooth muscle relaxation. The intestinal smooth muscle relaxation is initiated by an alpha$_2$-adrenergic receptor.

445–449. The answers are: 445-B, 446-C, 447-A, 448-B, 449-A. *(Ganong, 15/e. pp 207–213.)* The autonomic nervous system, consisting of two divisions—sympathetic and parasympathetic—controls the primarily involuntary visceral functions of the body. It is activated essentially by centers in the spinal cord, brainstem, and hypothalamus with modulation by input from cortical or limbic centers. The afferent portion of the system consists of specialized receptors sensitive to, for example, pressure, temperature, pH, and osmotic pressure. Their cell bodies are located in spinal dorsal roots or cranial nerve ganglia, and they convey impulses via sympathetic and parasympathetic pathways. The peripheral motor portions of the system consist of preganglionic and postganglionic neurons. The preganglionic neurons are located in the spinal cord and in the motor nuclei of the cranial nerves.

The sympathetic division of the autonomic nervous system is located primarily in the thoracic and lumbar regions, whereas the parasympathetic division is confined to the brainstem and sacral region. Sympathetic preganglionic fibers end on the cell bodies of their postganglionic neurons. These postganglionic neurons are localized in a series of discrete paravertebral ganglia and in several large peripheral ganglia, e.g., the celiac and mesenteric ganglia. Fibers may synapse at the same level as their respective cell bodies or pass upward or downward for several levels before reaching their postganglionic sites. Parasympathetic preganglionic fibers from the cranial division proceed almost exclusively via the vagus nerve to synapse with postganglionic cell bodies located in or near the visceral structures they supply.

The preganglionic fibers of both systems are cholinergic; i.e., they secrete acetylcholine at their synaptic terminals. Parasympathetic postganglionic fibers are also cholinergic, whereas sympathetic postganglionic fibers are primarily noradrenergic; i.e., they secrete norepinephrine. However, sympathetic fibers that innervate sweat glands and skeletal muscle arterioles are cholinergic.

The sympathetic and parasympathetic systems are both capable of exerting excitatory and inhibitory actions and often oppose each other. In general, most organs are controlled dominantly by one or the other.

450–454. The answers are: 450-B, 451-B, 452-A, 453-A, 454-A. *(Ganong, 15/e. pp 115–121.)* The Golgi tendon organ (GTO) is connected in series with the muscle, whereas the muscle spindle is in parallel. As a result of this anatomic arrangement, the muscle spindle is stretched when the muscle is stretched and becomes slack when the muscle is contracted. In contrast, the GTO is stretched when the muscle is contracted. Thus the activity generated by the GTO is proportional to the amount of force generated by the muscle, whereas the activity of the muscle spindle is proportional to the amount of stretch placed on the muscle. Although the GTOs are stretched slightly when a muscle is stretched, this is not usually enough to cause an increase in GTO activity. If not coactivated by the gamma motoneurons, the muscle spindles will stop firing during a muscle contraction. If, however, the gamma motoneurons do fire, this will prevent cessation of activity during a contraction or, if the muscle is at rest, will cause an increase in muscle spindle activity. GTOs are not affected by the gamma motoneurons. The Ia afferents from muscle spindles cause the muscle to contract via a monosynaptic pathway. The Ib afferents from the GTOs cause the muscle to relax through a disynaptic pathway.

455–458. The answers are: 455-A, 456-B, 457-D, 458-B. *(Ganong, 15/e. pp 137–139.)* The visual pathway consists of the retina, optic nerve, optic chiasma, optic tract, and visual (or occipital) cerebral cortex, in that order. The spatial relationships of fibers in the retina are maintained in the pattern of fibers leaving the eye via the optic nerve: fibers representing the temporal retina (nasal field) stay on the same side and fibers representing the nasal retina (temporal field) cross at the optic chiasma.

Defects in the field of vision can result from primary diseases of the retina or interruption of the optic pathway. Defects caused by primary retinal disease or vascular disease (hypertension or diabetes) often begin at the periphery of vision and may produce numerous small defects, or scotomata. Visual field analysis can be employed to localize lesions in the optic pathway that are causing blindness. Thus, a lesion involving the optic chiasma will block impulses from the nasal halves of both retinae to produce bitemporal hemianopia (choice B in the question). Such lesions are most commonly caused by pituitary tumors. The pituitary gland is situated in the sella turcica immediately beneath the optic chiasma, from which it is separated by a dural membrane, the diaphragma sellae. Enlargement of the pituitary by tumor or infiltrative processes frequently results in upward expansion, causing compression of the optic chiasma and interruption of the decussating fibers from the nasal retinae.

Interruption of one optic nerve will clearly produce total blindness in the affected eye (choice A). Besides trauma, other processes that may cause optic nerve deficits include orbital tumors or compromise of the blood supply.

Interruption of an optic tract beyond the optic chiasma would denervate the half of the retina on the same side as the lesion and produce a contralateral visual defect referred to as homonymous hemianopia (choice D). The defect illustrated in choice C, in which there is loss of nasal fields bilaterally, could not occur from a lesion at a single site.

459–460. The answers are: 459-C, 460-C. *(Berne, 2/e. pp 28–29, 32–38.)* The driving force for an ion is the sum of the electrical and diffusional forces acting on the ion. The driving force is calculated from the formula $E_M - E_{ion}$, where E_M is the membrane potential and E_{ion} is the Nernst, or equilibrium, potential for the ion. Based on this formula, the driving force for an ion is greatest when the difference between the membrane potential and the equilibrium potential for that ion is greatest. Since E_K (equilibrium potential for potassium) is -92 mV, the driving force is greatest when the membrane is most positive. In this case, this is at point C. The upstroke of the action potential is caused by an increase in sodium conductance. Sodium conductance begins to increase at threshold (point B) and reaches a maximum near the peak of the action potential (point C). Points B through D are part of the absolute refractory period. During this period, a second action potential cannot occur. Point E is part of the relative refractory period. During this period a second action potential can be generated, but the stimulus strength must be greater than normal. When the net ionic fluxes across a membrane are zero, the membrane potential is not changing. Such a situation occurs when the cell is at the resting potential (point A) and at the peaks of the overshoot and undershoot.

Cellular Physiology

DIRECTIONS: Each question below contains five suggested responses. Select the **one best** response to each question.

461. Which of the following characteristics of an axon is most dependent on its diameter?

(A) Its resting potential
(B) The duration of its refractory period
(C) The conduction velocity of its action potential
(D) The overshoot of its action potential
(E) The activity of its sodium-potassium pump

462. The resting potential of a nerve membrane is primarily dependent on the concentration gradient of

(A) potassium
(B) sodium
(C) calcium
(D) chloride
(E) bicarbonate

463. Which of the following solutions has the greatest osmolality?

(A) 100 mM glucose
(B) 100 mM sodium chloride
(C) 75 mM calcium chloride
(D) 75 mM urea
(E) None of the above; they all have the same osmolality

464. If the extracellular concentration of a substance doubles from 10 mM to 20 mM while the intracellular concentration remains at 5 mM, the rate of diffusion increases

(A) twofold
(B) threefold
(C) fourfold
(D) fivefold
(E) tenfold

465. Which of the following statements best characterizes a molecule whose reflection coefficient to a membrane is zero?

(A) It will not permeate the membrane
(B) It can only cross the membrane through the lipid bilayer
(C) It causes water to flow across the membrane
(D) It is as diffusible through the membrane as water
(E) It is transported across the membrane by a carrier

466. The characteristic of a water-insoluble substance most important in governing its diffusibility through a cell membrane is its

(A) hydrated diameter
(B) molecular weight
(C) electrical charge
(D) lipid solubility
(E) three-dimensional shape

467. Which one of the following muscle proteins plays an important role in contraction of both smooth and striated muscle?

(A) Calmodulin
(B) Troponin
(C) Tropomyosin
(D) Actin
(E) Myosin light chains

468. During the process of excitation-contraction coupling in smooth muscle, calcium is released from the sarcoplasmic reticulum by

(A) inositol triphosphate (IP_3)
(B) protein kinase C
(C) diacyl glycerol (DAG)
(D) cyclic AMP (cAMP)
(E) calmodulin

469. Which of the following words or phrases is most closely associated with an end-plate potential at the neuromuscular junction?

(A) "All-or-none response"
(B) Depolarization
(C) Hyperpolarization
(D) Membrane propagation
(E) Electrically excitable gates

470. In a nerve, the magnitude of the action potential overshoot is normally a function of the

(A) magnitude of the stimulus
(B) intracellular potassium concentration
(C) extracellular sodium concentration
(D) resting membrane potential
(E) diameter of the axon

471. When circulating catecholamines bind to beta receptors on bronchiolar smooth muscle, their primary effect is caused by the

(A) opening of receptor-activated calcium channels
(B) release of calcium from the sarcoplasmic reticulum
(C) phosphorylation of intracellular proteins
(D) depolarization of the cell membrane
(E) activation of troponin C

472. Which of the following is an important component of excitation-contraction coupling in both smooth and skeletal muscle?

(A) The inward flow of calcium across the muscle membrane
(B) The binding of myosin cross-bridges to actin filaments
(C) The binding of calcium to troponin
(D) The phosphorylation of myosin
(E) The depolarization of the muscle membrane

473. Which of the following statements about impulse transmission in the normal myoneural junction is true?

(A) It is stimulated by high levels of cholinesterase
(B) It is associated with an influx of potassium ions through the muscle membrane
(C) It is depressed by abnormally low levels of magnesium
(D) It is unaffected by extremely high rates of stimulation of the nerve fiber
(E) It is dependent upon the amount of acetylcholine released at the end-plate

474. When comparing the contractile responses in smooth and skeletal muscle, which of the following factors is most different?

(A) The source of activator calcium
(B) The role of calcium in initiating contraction
(C) The mechanism of force generation
(D) The source of energy used during contraction
(E) The nature of the contractile proteins

475. The generation of excitation-contraction coupling involves all the following events EXCEPT

(A) generation of end-plate potential
(B) release of calcium from troponin
(C) formation of cross-linkages between actin and myosin
(D) depolarization along transverse tubules
(E) hydrolysis of ATP to ADP

476. The amount of tension that a whole muscle can produce is greatest in which of the following situations?

(A) In the single twitch response
(B) During maximal incomplete tetanus
(C) During submaximal complete tetanus
(D) During maximal complete tetanus
(E) When all the fibers are excited by a single stimulus pulse

477. The "all-or-none law" of nerve fibers states that

(A) the impulse initiated by a strong stimulus is conducted more rapidly than the impulse initiated by a weaker stimulus
(B) the impulse initiated by a strong stimulus is stronger than the impulse initiated by a weaker stimulus
(C) the stimulus that just exceeds the threshold for excitation of a nerve causes as strong an impulse as a stimulus twice as great
(D) weak stimuli capable of initiating an impulse depolarize less of the nerve surface than stronger stimuli
(E) either all or none of the potassium in a nerve cell passes out through the membrane when an impulse passes

478. True statements about the sarcoplasmic reticulum include which of the following?

(A) It is necessary for propagation of an action potential along the muscle membrane
(B) It is continuous with the sarcolemma
(C) It is rich in mitochondria
(D) It catalyzes the calcium-dependent hydrolysis of ATP
(E) It is responsible for maintaining the resting membrane potential

479. Correct comparisons between fast- and slow-twitch skeletal muscle fibers include all the following EXCEPT

(A) fast-twitch fibers fatigue more rapidly
(B) fast-twitch fibers develop more force
(C) fast-twitch fibers store more glycogen
(D) fast-twitch fibers require a higher frequency of stimulation to produce tetanus
(E) fast-twitch fibers contain a higher concentration of mitochondria

480. The velocity of nerve conduction is increased with a decrease in the

(A) diameter of the nerve fiber
(B) degree of myelinization
(C) space constant of the nerve fiber
(D) capacitance of the nerve fiber membrane
(E) resting membrane potential

481. The rate of diffusion of a particle across a membrane will increase if

(A) the area of the membrane decreases
(B) the thickness of the membrane increases
(C) the size of the particle increases
(D) the concentration gradient of the particle decreases
(E) the lipid solubility of the particle increases

482. Simple and facilitated diffusion are alike in that both

(A) display saturation kinetics
(B) require some sort of carrier mechanism for transport
(C) can work in the absence of ATP
(D) can transport material against a concentration gradient
(E) can be blocked by specific inhibitors

483. The flow of calcium into the cell is an important component of the upstroke phase of action potentials in

(A) cardiac ventricular muscle
(B) intestinal smooth muscle
(C) skeletal muscle fibers
(D) nerve cell bodies
(E) none of the above

484. The membrane potential will depolarize by the greatest amount if the membrane permeability increases for

(A) potassium
(B) sodium and potassium
(C) chloride
(D) potassium and chloride
(E) sodium, potassium, and chloride

485. Which of the following will be less during the overshoot of an action potential than during the resting state?

(A) Membrane conductance for sodium
(B) Membrane conductance for potassium
(C) Transference for sodium
(D) Transference for potassium
(E) Total membrane conductance

486. If the membrane conductances for sodium and potassium are equal, the membrane potential is close to

(A) −90 mV
(B) −70 mV
(C) −15 mV
(D) 0 mV
(E) +40 mV

487. The flow of water in an osmotic pressure gradient is correctly described by all the following statements EXCEPT

(A) there is a net flow of water from a region of low osmotic pressure to one of a higher osmotic pressure
(B) the rate of water flow increases as the hydraulic conductivity increases
(C) there is a net flow of water from a region of low concentration of solute to a region of highly concentrated solute
(D) the rate of water flow increases as the reflection coefficient increases
(E) free energy is required for the flow of water

488. Statements descriptive of both the equilibrium and steady states include which of the following?

(A) The sum of all the fluxes across the membrane is zero in both
(B) Both are maintained by the consumption of free energy
(C) The concentration gradient across the membrane is zero in both
(D) Both are maintained by homeostatic processes
(E) The membrane potential is zero in both

489. During the relative refractory period

(A) the rate of depolarization is decreased
(B) the rate of repolarization is increased
(C) the threshold for eliciting an action potential is decreased
(D) the conductance of potassium is decreased
(E) the magnitude of the overshoot is increased

490. An increase in sodium conductance is associated with

(A) the plateau phase of the ventricular muscle action potential
(B) the downstroke of the skeletal muscle action potential
(C) the upstroke of the smooth muscle action potential
(D) the refractory period of the nerve cell action potential
(E) the end-plate potential of the skeletal muscle fiber

491. Electrically excitable gates are normally involved in

(A) the depolarization of the end-plate membrane by ACh
(B) hyperpolarization of the rods by light
(C) release of calcium from ventricular muscle sarcoplasmic reticulum
(D) transport of glucose into cells by a sodium-dependent, secondary active transport system
(E) increase in nerve cell potassium conductance caused by an increase in extracellular potassium

492. The sodium gradient across the nerve cell membrane is

(A) a result of the Donnan equilibrium
(B) significantly changed during an action potential
(C) used as a source of energy for the transport of other ions
(D) an important determinant of the resting membrane potential
(E) maintained by an Na-Ca exchanger

493. Increasing the extracellular potassium concentration will

(A) increase the threshold for eliciting an action potential
(B) hyperpolarize the membrane potential
(C) decrease potassium permeability
(D) decrease the activity of the sodium-potassium pump
(E) do none of the above

494. Which of the following would cause an immediate reduction in the amount of potassium leaking out of a cell?

(A) Increasing the permeability of the membrane to potassium
(B) Increasing the intracellular potassium concentration
(C) Increasing (hyperpolarizing) the membrane potential
(D) Reducing the activity of the sodium-potassium pump
(E) Decreasing the potassium equilibrium potential

495. Excitation-contraction coupling in smooth muscle is initiated when calcium binds to

(A) myosin light chains
(B) calmodulin
(C) troponin
(D) tropomyosin
(E) protein kinase A

496. All the following transport processes require energy EXCEPT the movement of

(A) sodium out of nerve cells
(B) calcium into the sarcoplasmic reticulum
(C) hydrogen into the lumen of the distal nephron
(D) glucose into adipose tissue
(E) potassium into striated muscle cells

DIRECTIONS: The group of questions below consists of four lettered headings followed by a set of numbered items. For each numbered item select

A   if the item is associated with   (A) **only**
B   if the item is associated with   (B) **only**
C   if the item is associated with   **both** (A) and (B)
D   if the item is associated with   **neither** (A) nor (B)

Each lettered heading may be used **once, more than once, or not at all.**

Questions 497–500

(A) Skeletal muscle
(B) Cardiac muscle
(C) Both
(D) Neither

497. Contractile force is varied by varying the amount of calcium released from the sarcoplasmic reticulum

498. Contractile force is varied by varying the preload

499. Contractile force is varied by varying the number of muscle fibers activated

500. Contractile force is varied by summation or tetanus

Cellular Physiology
Answers

461. The answer is C. *(West, 12/e. pp 41–45.)* The conduction velocity of an action potential along an axon is proportional to the axon's diameter for both unmyelinated and myelinated axons. In myelinated axons, the conduction velocity of an action potential also increases as the distance between nodes of Ranvier increases. The resting potential and the action potential of a nerve axon are dependent on the type and density of electrically excitable gates and the ability of the Na,K-ATPase to establish and maintain the concentration gradients. These characteristics are not related in any systematic way to the axon diameter.

462. The answer is A. *(West, 12/e. pp 36–38.)* The membrane potential is determined by the concentration gradient of the ion to which it is most permeable or for which it has the greatest conductance. In the resting state, the conductance for potassium is approximately nine times as great as the conductance for sodium. Hence, the membrane potential is dependent on the concentration gradient for potassium. The concentration gradient for chloride is not an important determinant of the membrane potential (even in those cells where chloride conductance is high) because, unlike sodium and potassium, which are actively pumped across the membrane, chloride is passively distributed across the membrane.

463. The answer is C. *(Berne, 2/e. pp 12–14.)* Osmolality is defined as the concentration of particles in solution. Thus, to determine the osmolality of a particular solution, you must first find out how many particles are formed from each molecule. Glucose and urea each yields 1 particle per mole, sodium chloride yields 2 particles per mole, and calcium chloride yields 3 particles per mole. The osmolality of the calcium chloride solution is thus higher (3 × 75 = 225) than the osmolality of the sodium chloride solution (2 × 100 = 200).

464. The answer is B. *(Guyton, 8/e. pp 43–44.)* According to Fick's law of diffusion, the rate of diffusion (flux) is proportional to the difference in concentration between the inside (Cin) and outside (Cout) of the membrane: Flux = P (Cin − Cout). In the example given, initially this difference was 10 mM − 5 mM, or 5 mM. With the change in extracellular concentration, the difference became 20 mM − 5 mM, or 15 mM. Since the concentration difference increased threefold (from 5 to 15), the rate of diffusion also increased threefold.

465. The answer is D. *(Berne, 2/e. pp 12–14.)* The reflection coefficient is a measure of a membrane's permeability to a substance in comparison to its permeability in water. It can be calculated from the following equation:

$$\text{Reflection coefficient} = \frac{P(\text{water}) - P(\text{substance})}{P(\text{water})}$$

It is also a measure of the actual osmotic pressure developed by the substance compared with the osmotic pressure it should theoretically develop according to Van't Hoff's equation. A substance with a reflection coefficient of zero would have the same diffusibility through the membrane as water and would not develop any osmotic pressure.

466. The answer is D. *(Berne, 2/e. pp 8–12.)* Materials that are not soluble in water can only cross the membrane through the lipid bilayer. The most important factor determining how well a substance can diffuse across the lipid bilayer is the substance's lipid solubility. If two materials have the same lipid solubility, then the diffusion coefficient of the smaller particle will be greater.

467. The answer is D. *(Berne, 2/e. pp 316–322, 325–326, 328–331.)* In excitation-contraction coupling in striated muscle, calcium initiates contraction by binding to troponin. The calcium-activated troponin then acts to remove the tropomyosin-mediated inhibition of actin-myosin interaction. In excitation-contraction coupling in smooth muscle, calcium initiates contraction by binding to calmodulin. The calcium-activated calmodulin then acts as a protein kinase, phosphorylating the myosin light chains. Actin-myosin interaction follows light-chain phosphorylation. In both smooth and striated muscle, the thin filaments are composed of actin.

468. The answer is A. *(Berne, 2/e. pp 682–683.)* The release of calcium from the sarcoplasmic reticulum in many smooth muscles is mediated by IP_3. When a calcium-mobilizing stimulus binds to its receptor on the cell membrane, it activates a phosphatase enzyme, phospholipase C. The phospholipase C cleaves inositol diphosphate (a membrane-bound lipid) into IP_3 and DAG. IP_3 causes the release of calcium from the sarcoplasmic reticulum. DAG activates protein kinase C, whose function is not well understood.

469. The answer is B. *(Guyton, 8/e. pp 81–83.)* An end-plate potential is a depolarization caused by the opening of chemically excitable gates in response to the release of acetylcholine from the presynaptic nerve terminals of alpha motoneurons. Its magnitude is proportional to the amount of transmitter released. Although it is not propagated, it acts as a stimulus for the generation of an action potential on the muscle membrane contiguous to the end-plate region. The action potential is propagated and results in a muscle twitch.

470. The answer is C. *(Guyton, 8/e. pp 55–58.)* An action potential is normally an all-or-none response; that is, its magnitude is independent of the stimulus strength. The magnitude of the action potential is reduced during the relative refractory period or when the membrane is depolarized by an abnormally high extracellular potassium concentration. However, the upstroke of the action potential is caused by an inward flow of sodium ions, and thus its magnitude depends on the extracellular sodium concentration.

471. The answer is C. *(Berne, 2/e. pp 336, 682–683.)* When norepinephrine, epinephrine, or exogenously administered catecholamines bind to beta receptors, they activate a guanyl nucleotide-binding protein called the G_s (or N_s) protein. The activated G protein in turn activates adenylate cyclase, which catalyzes the conversion of ATP into cyclic AMP (cAMP). The cAMP then activates a protein kinase (cAMP-dependent protein kinase). The protein kinase phosphorylates a variety of intracellular and membrane proteins that produce the relaxation of bronchiolar smooth muscle observed in response to adrenergic agonist stimulation.

472. The answer is B. *(Berne, 2/e. pp 327–331. Ganong, 15/e. p 61.)* Excitation-contraction coupling in skeletal muscle requires membrane depolarization and the binding of calcium to troponin. In contrast, smooth muscle can contract in the absence of membrane depolarization (by a process called *pharmacomechanical coupling*) and does not contain troponin. Smooth muscle contraction is initiated by cross-bridge phosphorylation. In skeletal muscle calcium is derived exclusively from the sarcoplasmic reticulum, whereas in smooth muscle a significant portion of the calcium comes from the extracellular fluid. Contraction in both is due to the sliding of the thin (actin) filaments across the thick (myosin) filaments brought about by the binding of myosin cross-bridges to the actin filaments.

473. The answer is E. *(West, 12/e. pp 59–60.)* Impulse transmission at the myoneural junction depends on the release of acetylcholine. High levels of cholinesterase would tend to interfere with transmission, as would high (not low) levels of magnesium. The release of acetylcholine at the myoneural junction is thought to be associated with an influx of calcium ions into the terminal membranes. Extremely rapid rates of stimulation cause depletion of acetylcholine stores and would result in fatigue of the myoneural junction.

474. The answer is B. *(Berne, 2/e. pp 331–336.)* In both smooth and skeletal muscle, force is generated by the cycling of cross-bridges. ATP provides the energy for the cycling of the cross-bridges in both muscles. In skeletal muscle, activator calcium comes exclusively from the sarcoplasmic reticulum (SR), while in smooth muscle calcium can come both from the SR and from the extracellular fluid. However, the greatest difference in excitation-contraction coupling involves the role of calcium in initiating contraction. In smooth muscle, calcium binds to and activates calmodulin, which acts as a kinase to catalyze the phosphorylation of the 20,000-dalton myosin light chain (LC_{20}). Once the light chains are phosphorylated, myosin cross-bridges bind to actin on the thin filaments, which initiates contraction. In skeletal muscle, calcium binds to troponin, which removes the tropomyosin-mediated inhibition of the actin-myosin interactions. Once the inhibition is removed, cross-bridge cycling (and contraction) begins.

475. The answer is B. *(Ganong, 15/e. pp 61–62.)* In excitation-contraction coupling, depolarization of the muscle fiber follows generation of the endplate potential. The depolarization is transmitted via the transverse tubule system into the inner portion of the muscle fiber, where it triggers release of calcium from sarcoplasmic reticulum. Calcium binds to troponin C, which permits formation of cross-linkages between actin and myosin and sliding of thin and thick filaments. Reaccumulation of calcium by sarcoplasmic reticulum followed by release of calcium from troponin results in cessation of actin-myosin interaction and relaxation.

476. The answer is D. *(Ganong, 15/e. p 63.)* The single muscle twitch generates only a single, sudden contraction. During summation, individual muscle twitches are added together to make strong muscle movements. Indeed, the tension developed during summation is much greater than during the single muscle twitch. When a muscle is stimulated at progressively greater frequencies, activation of the contractile mechanism occurs repeatedly before any relaxation has occurred and the successive contractions fuse into one continuous contraction. Such a response is called *tetanus*. During complete tetanus there is no relaxation between stimuli; during incomplete tetanus there are periods of incomplete relaxation between the summated stimuli. The tension developed during complete tetanus is about four times that developed by the individual twitch contractions.

477. The answer is C. *(Ganong, 15/e. p 48.)* The all-or-none law of nerve fibers states that a nerve fiber can respond in only a single way. Thus, *any* stimulus capable of depolarizing a given nerve fiber will result in the *same* impulse, however much the intensity of the stimulus may exceed the threshold intensity. It should be observed that this law applies to single nerve fibers and not to nerve bundles, where differing stimuli can have differing end results because of variations in the number of individual nerve fibers stimulated.

478. The answer is D. *(Berne, 2/e. pp 329–336.)* The sarcoplasmic reticulum is a complex tubular organelle, distinct from the mitochondria, that forms a network parallel to the myofilaments and terminates in terminal cisterns at each end of the sarcomere. Its primary function is to release calcium into the cytoplasm surrounding the myofilaments during contraction and to sequester calcium during relaxation. Sequestration of calcium is accomplished by the action of a membrane-bound active transport protein that uses ATP and transports calcium against a concentration gradient. The terminal cisterns of the sarcoplasmic reticulum lie adjacent to the transverse, or T, tubules, which are continuous with the sarcolemma or plasma membrane and facilitate transmission of the action potential from the neuromuscular junction to the interior of the muscle fiber.

479. The answer is E. *(Berne, 2/e. pp 348–351.)* Fast-twitch fibers are characterized by their large size, high capacity for anaerobic metabolism, high development of force, high speed of contraction, and short twitch times. They are unable to replenish their ATP supply quickly because they are relatively poorly perfused and have few mitochondria; this results in rapid fatigue. They are able to sustain contraction for a short time because of their relatively large (compared with those of slow-twitch fibers) glycogen stores. They have a short duration of contraction because their SR calcium pumps rapidly resequester calcium. In order for summation or tetanus to occur, a second stimulus must be applied before the muscle relaxes. The shorter the duration of contraction, the more frequently the muscle must be stimulated to produce tetanus.

480. The answer is D. *(Berne, 2/e. pp 41–45.)* In order for propagation of an action potential to occur the depolarization produced by one action potential must depolarize the adjacent patch of excitable membrane to threshold. The amount of charge that must flow to produce this depolarization varies inversely with the membrane capacitance. Thus, as the capacitance decreases, the velocity of conduction increases. The rate of charge flow decreases as the diameter of the nerve fiber decreases, thus decreasing the velocity of conduction. The space constant ($\sqrt{R_m/R_{in}}$) is a measure of how far along the axon the charge will flow. The degree of myelinization determines the magnitude of the membrane resistance (R_m); thus, when myelinization decreases, membrane resistance decreases and the space constant decreases. Velocity of conduction decreases as the space constant decreases. Decreasing the resting membrane potential inactivates sodium channels. This will decrease the flow of charge across the membrane during an action potential and thus decrease the velocity of propagation.

481. The answer is E. *(West, 12/e. pp 17–19.)* The rate of diffusion is described by Fick's law, which states that the flux of material across a membrane is directly proportional to the area of a membrane and the concentration difference of the particles on either side of the membrane and is inversely proportional to the thickness of the membrane. In general, if all other properties of the membrane are the same, the larger the particle the more difficulty it will have crossing the membrane. Similarly, for a particle to cross a membrane, it must first dissolve in the membrane. For lipid-soluble substances, the greater the lipid solubility, the greater the amount dissolved in the membrane and the greater the flux.

482. The answer is C. *(West, 12/e. pp 17–19, 21–22.)* Neither simple nor facilitated diffusion requires free energy to transport material across a membrane, so both can function in the absence of ATP. Because they do not use free energy, neither can transport material against a concentration gradient. Facilitated diffusion is a carrier-mediated process and so displays saturation kinetics and can be blocked by specific inhibitory substances that bind to the carrier.

483. The answer is B. *(Berne, 2/e. pp 34–35, 39–40, 653–655.)* In cells of the cardiac ventricular muscle, the plateau phase of the action potential, but not the upstroke, is accompanied by the flow of calcium into the cells. In intestinal smooth muscle, the upstroke of the action potential is caused by the flow of calcium into the cell. Skeletal muscle fibers resemble nerve fibers. In both of these cells, the upstroke of the action potential is caused by the flow of sodium into the cell.

484. The answer is B. *(West, 12/e. pp 35–38.)* When the permeability of a particular ion is increased, the membrane potential moves toward the equilibrium potential for that ion. The equilibrium potentials for chloride (-80 mV) and potassium (-92 mV) are close to the resting membrane potential, so increases in their permeability have little effect on the resting membrane potential. The equilibrium potential for sodium ($+60$ mV) is very far from the resting membrane potential. Thus, increasing the permeability for sodium causes a large depolarization. When the increase in sodium permeability is combined with an increase in potassium permeability, the amount of depolarization produced is greater than that produced when sodium, potassium, and chloride permeabilities are all increased.

485. The answer is D. *(West, 12/e. pp 35–38, 47–51.)* During an action potential the conductance for both sodium and potassium is higher than it is at rest. However, the conductance for sodium is higher than the conductance for potassium during the overshoot. Hence, the transference for potassium is less. Recall that transference is a measure of an ion's relative conductance:

$$\text{Transference (ion)} = \frac{\text{Conductance (ion)}}{\text{Total conductance}}$$

486. The answer is C. *(West, 12/e. pp 37–38.)* The membrane potential can be calculated using the equivalent circuit analysis based on the principle that the net current flow through the membrane at rest is zero. According to the equivalent circuit analysis, $E_M =$

$$\frac{(E_K \times g_K) + (E_{Na} \times g_{Na})}{g_K + g_{Na}}$$

Solving this equation when $g_K = g_{Na}$ yields

$$\frac{-92 + {}+60}{2} = -16 \text{ mV}$$

487. The answer is E. *(Berne, 2/e. pp 12–15.)* The ability of dissolved particles to cause the flow of water across a membrane by osmosis increases when the permeability of the membrane to the particles decreases and increases when the hydraulic conductivity of the membrane to water increases. An increase in the reflection coefficient indicates that the permeability of the membrane to the particles is decreasing. The osmotic pressure is higher on the side of the membrane where the concentration of particles is higher, but, paradoxically, the osmotic flow of water is toward the side of the membrane that has the higher osmotic pressure.

488. The answer is A. *(West, 12/e. pp 14–18, 28–30.)* In both an equilibrium and a steady state condition, there is no change in the concentration of materials inside or outside the cell. However, in a steady state condition energy must be consumed to keep the concentrations from changing. An equilibrium condition is not considered to be a homeostatic process because active physiologic mechanisms are not used to maintain it. Membrane potential and concentration differences across the membrane can be maintained in both states.

489. The answer is A. *(Berne, 2/e. p 40.)* During the relative refractory period, an action potential can still be elicited, but the stimulus must be stronger than normal. The larger stimulus is required because the threshold is increased owing to the increases in potassium conductance and sodium inactivation that occur during the action potential. These changes in membrane permeability are also responsible for causing the decreases in the rate of rise and overshoot of the action potential that occur during the relative refractory period. The decrease in the overshoot potential causes a decrease in the number of potassium channels that open during the action potential. Thus the repolarization phase of the action potential is slower than normal.

490. The answer is E. *(Berne, 2/e. pp 34–35, 49–52, 331–336.)* The channel opened by ACh when it binds to receptors on the end plates of skeletal muscle fibers is equally permeable to potassium and sodium. The increase in sodium permeability allows sodium to flow into the cell and produces the end-plate potential. The plateau phase of ventricular muscle action potentials and the upstroke of smooth muscle action potentials are produced by an increase in calcium conductance. An increase in potassium conductance is responsible for the downstroke of the action potential. The refractory period is caused by an increase in potassium conductance and a decrease in the number of sodium channels available to produce an action potential (i.e., sodium channel inactivation).

491. The answer is E. *(Berne, 2/e. pp 49–50, 331–334, 399–401. Ganong, 15/e. pp 61–62. West, 12/e. pp 979–980.)* Electrically excitable gates are those that respond to a change in membrane potential. The most notable electrically excitable gates are those on the sodium and potassium channels that produce the nerve action potential. The potassium channel gate is opened by depolarization. When potassium is added to the extracellular fluid, it depolarizes the nerve cell membrane and causes the electrically excitable gates on the potassium channel to open. Ventricular muscle sarcoplasmic reticulum releases its calcium in response to an increase in intracellular calcium. In skeletal muscle, depolarization of the T tubule causes electrically driven calcium channels on the SR to open. The gates opened by ACh are chemically excitable gates. In rods, sodium channels are closed when cGMP is hydrolyzed. Glucose transport is not regulated by gates.

492. The answer is C. *(Berne, 2/e. pp 24–28.)* The sodium-potassium pump uses the energy contained in ATP to maintain the sodium gradient across the membrane. The sodium gradient, in turn, is used to transport other substances across the membrane. For example, the Na-Ca exchanger uses the energy in the sodium gradient to help maintain the low intracellular calcium required for normal cell function. Although sodium enters the cell during an action potential, the quantity of sodium is so small that no significant change in intracellular sodium concentration occurs. Because the sodium transference is so low, the sodium equilibrium potential is not an important determinant of the resting membrane potential.

493. The answer is A. *(Ganong, 15/e. pp 31–52.)* When the extracellular potassium concentration is increased, the membrane depolarizes. Depolarization causes potassium channels to open, which increases potassium permeability. Depolarization also causes sodium channels to inactivate, which reduces the number of sodium channels that are able to open in response to a stimulus. Since fewer channels can respond to the stimulus, a larger-than-normal stimulus is required to generate an action potential. The activity of the sodium-potassium pump may increase somewhat in response to the increase in extracellular potassium. However, the increase will be quite small because the potassium binding sites on the pump are nearly saturated at normal physiologic potassium concentrations.

494. The answer is C. *(Berne, 2/e. pp 26–29.)* The amount of potassium leaking out of the cell depends on its driving force and its membrane conductance. The driving force is the difference between the membrane potential and the equilibrium potential for potassium. Since the membrane potential is more positive than the equilibrium potential for potassium, hyperpolarizing the membrane (that is, making it more negative) would reduce the driving force. Increasing the intracellular potassium concentration increases the equilibrium potential for potassium, that is, makes it more negative and thus increases the driving force. Reducing the sodium-potassium pump activity would cause the potassium concentration gradient to fall, which, in turn, would cause a decrease in the amount of potassium leaking out of the cell. However, this would not occur immediately. In fact, because the pump is electrogenic, a small depolarization would initially follow a cessation of pump activity and this would cause an increase in the driving force for potassium.

495. The answer is B. *(Ganong, 15/e. pp 73–74.)* Smooth muscle contraction is regulated by a series of reactions that begins with the binding of calcium to calmodulin. The calcium-calmodulin complex then binds to and activates a protein kinase called *myosin light chain kinase (MLCK)*. MLCK catalyzes the phosphorylation of the myosin light chains (LC-20). Once these light chains are phosphorylated, myosin and actin interaction can occur and the muscle shortens and develops tension. Although two molecules of ATP are required to initiate contraction, one for the phosphorylation of myosin light chains and one to bend the myosin cross-bridge, smooth muscle is energetically efficient because the rate of cross-bridge cycling is so slow.

496. The answer is D. *(Ganong, 15/e. pp 29–30, 62, 316, 669.)* Glucose is transported into fat cells by facilitated diffusion and thus does not require the direct or indirect use of energy. Insulin increases the rate of diffusion but is not necessary for the diffusion. Sodium and potassium are transported by the Na-K pump, calcium is transported into the sarcoplasmic reticulum by a Ca pump, and hydrogen is transported by an H^+ pump. All of these transporters use ATP directly in the transport process. In the proximal tubule, hydrogen is secreted by an Na-H exchange process; this is an example of secondary active transport.

497–500. The answers are: 497-B, 498-C, 499-A, 500-A. *(Berne, 2/e. pp 322–326, 331–334.)* Under normal circumstances, the force of contraction of a skeletal muscle is varied by varying the preload, the number of motor units recruited, and the summation or tetanus. In the heart, all the muscle fibers must be activated during each contraction to eject the blood efficiently. Thus, the number of fibers recruited during each heart beat is always the same. In cardiac muscle, the durations of the action potential and contractile event are similar, so under normal circumstances, summation and tetanus cannot occur. The major mechanisms for varying contractile force in cardiac muscle are variations in preload and in the amount of activator calcium released from the sarcoplasmic reticulum (SR). However, in skeletal muscle the amount of calcium released from the SR is always sufficient to activate all the contractile proteins. Thus, skeletal muscle does not use variations in release of calcium from the SR to vary contractile force.

Bibliography

Berne RM, Levy MN: *Physiology,* 2/e. St. Louis, CV Mosby, 1988.

Ganong WF: *Review of Medical Physiology,* 15/e. East Norwalk, CT, Appleton & Lange, 1991.

Guyton, AC: *Textbook of Medical Physiology,* 8/e. Philadelphia, WB Saunders, 1991.

Rose BD: *Clinical Physiology of Acid-Base and Electrolyte Disorders,* 3/e. New York, McGraw-Hill, 1989.

West JB: *Best and Taylor's Physiological Basis of Medical Practice,* 12/e. Baltimore, Williams & Wilkins, 1990.